LIVING LONGER

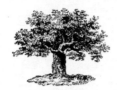

WORKING STRONGER

Dr. Kevin Fosnocht

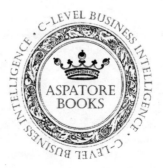

Published by Aspatore, Inc.

Please help us make this book better by emailing us corrections, updates, comments or any other inquiries at info@aspatore.com.

First Printing, 2003
10 9 8 7 6 5 4 3 2 1

ISBN 1-58762-356-0

Cover design by Traci Whitney

Material in this book is for informational purposes only. Please consult a doctor before trying any of the recommendations in this book you are not comfortable assuming personal liability for. The author and the publisher assume no liability for any actions performed as a result of this book.

This book is printed on acid free paper.

A special thanks to all the individuals that made this book possible.

About ASPATORE – Publishers of C-Level Business Intelligence
www.Aspatore.com

Aspatore Books is the largest and most exclusive publisher of C-Level executives (CEO, CFO, CTO, CMO, Partner) from the world's most respected companies. Aspatore annually publishes a select group of C-Level executives from the Global 1,000, top 250 professional services firms, law firms (Partners & Chairs), and other leading companies of all sizes. C-Level Business Intelligence ™, as conceptualized and developed by Aspatore Books, provides professionals of all levels with proven business intelligence from industry insiders – direct and unfiltered insight from those who know it best – as opposed to third-party accounts offered by unknown authors and analysts. Aspatore Books is committed to publishing a highly innovative line of business books, and redefining such resources as indispensable tools for all professionals.

LIVING LONGER
WORKING STRONGER

TABLE OF CONTENTS

CHAPTER 1
SURVIVING AND THRIVING

This book challenges you to look at your health as an important item on your personal balance sheet. Believing your health to be a "sure thing" asset, without regularly assessing its value, can eventually risk that very asset becoming a real liability.

Most business professionals are familiar with and regularly review "profit and loss" statements. Such a real-time assessment of the financial well-being of a company provides the information necessary for executives to make decisions that will not only insure that the business survives—but, perhaps more importantly, that it thrives. This book contains information that will allow you to perform such an assessment of your own health—and strategize to a thriving life.

It is impossible to read the newspaper, listen to the radio, or watch television, without being bombarded with the word "healthy." One cannot go shopping, to the grocery store, or out to eat without confronting the term. Through all kinds of media we are encouraged, persuaded, even enticed, to *be* healthy. The images conjured by the term—or at least the images we now associate with the word "healthy"—are usually pictures of young, thin, muscular, tanned people having fun in the sun with other young, thin, muscular, tanned people. It is certainly no accident that these same types of people are used to promote unhealthy behaviors like cigarette smoking and alcohol drinking.

We use the word "healthy" to convey a description of something, such as food (like fruits and vegetables) or an activity (like exercise). But we also use the term to convey a judgment. "Healthy" refers to something inherently good; "unhealthy" to something bad. Consider how we use the word to describe an attitude. One might say, "She has a very healthy outlook on the whole situation." In this context, the word "healthy" conveys a meaning of at least adaptation, if not strength or resilience.

What does the word "healthy" mean? The noun "health" comes from the Indo-European word *kailo*. From this root word come many other terms, which, I will argue in this book, are linked in ways that provide us with a schema, or map, to live *healthy* lives. Consider these terms for a moment, pausing to reflect on their connection to what you mean when you use the term "healthy:"

Whole
Wholesome
Heal
Holy

Over time, western technological thinking has fractured the meaning of the term "healthy." Our society has separated the physical, the emotional, the rational, and the spiritual from each other. An example of this separation can be seen in product marketing, which would lead us to believe that *things* are healthy: the right foods, the right drinks, the right supplements, the right exercise machine. I will argue that just as health can be ascribed only to living organisms, and for our discussion that refers to human beings, so too can the term healthy be ascribed only to behavior—not things. This proper emphasis carries with it a challenge to the reader: behavior—your behavior—is what is healthy or unhealthy. Though this book will provide important information about food, nutrition, activity, even tests and medications that modern medicine offers, the bottom line is that health—wholeness, healing—is the result of what you do—your choices, your behavior.

Health, then, is not simply the absence of disease. Implied in the term is a sense of fullness, of vitality, of realized potential. Most of our standards for health as a society, however, are determined by measuring the presence or absence of disease. It is quite intuitive and very logical to consider the health of a population in terms of disease states. A disease state is identifiable and its frequency in a population is measurable. We also use life-expectancy or longevity as an indicator of health. This too makes sense: Disease can end life and the shorter the average life-span of a population, the less "healthy" that population would be considered to be.

We will review the basic health statistics, as measured by life expectancy and disease status, of our country's population, but ultimately, as we consider you the business professional, our focus will primarily be on not only what choices you make, but how and why those choices are made. Though longevity and prevention or avoidance of disease are important goals for one who wants to lead a healthy life, it is very likely that you the reader are interested in more than simply surviving. I would argue that you are reading this book not only so that you might *survive*—but also that you might *thrive*.

Every day in my primary care internal medicine practice I see business professionals who are indeed surviving. Many have considerable health problems which medicines and other treatments are able to control but not cure. A significant amount of their personal and financial resources are bound up in surviving. Most of our office time together is spent in identifying and planning further survival techniques: how to minimize the effects of a medication I have prescribed, how to make their chronic pain more tolerable, how to make decisions on what next diagnostic or therapeutic intervention might be necessary. I certainly contribute to their health, if by that we mean longevity or the control or management of disease, but I often question—as I'm sure my patients do—whether I am helping them be healthy.

There are scores of books, magazines, and web sites devoted to the "mind-body connection." Though the term has nearly entered the vernacular, it is my experience as a physician that most people do not readily accept the fundamental premise underlying the concept. What's more, most people do not consider their health in the context of the meaning of the mind-body connection. And even fewer people bring this understanding into their doctors' offices when they discuss health concerns. So, there is an apparent disparity between the popularity of the mind-body connection concept and the number of people who actually employ the concept and its implications in their lives.

Let's take a moment to explore what is meant by the term "mind-body" connection. The term implies first and foremost that the mind and body are not separate; that they are not clearly divisible or distinct from one another; that we cannot "find" the mind in a delimited way; that the mind is bound to the body; the two are connected. The underlying premise is that those aspects of our selves that we traditionally call "the mind," such as thoughts and beliefs, are not only *connected* to the body but *affect* the body. The converse is also implied: The body affects the mind. The mind and the body are bound in a dynamic interplay.

The fundamental premise underlying the concept of the mind-body connection is that our bodies (heart, blood, bones, muscles, nerves, and brain) and our minds (thoughts and beliefs) profoundly affect, influence, and, in some cases, create each other. Let us start with our own thoughts. We can certainly identify these thoughts as such, but we know they are dependent on, or manufactured by, the functions of our anatomy and physiology: some*thing* (like the brain) has to function in a particular way to *do* the thinking. Most of us are comfortable with this mechanistic view. It proposes a "one-way" flow of information: The brain—through neurochemistry—creates thoughts. But the premise of the "mind-body connection" does not stop with the assertion that thoughts are simply the product of our anatomy and physiology. Such an assertion reduces our thoughts and emotions—and, some would have it, our entire consciousness—to a mere byproduct of physiology. The mind-body connection premise presents a more dynamic, complex, and, I believe, accurate understanding of the self. Not only does the body participate in the creation of thoughts, but our thoughts can directly affect the body. The mind and body are truly interdependent and involved in a complex interplay.

The dramatic interplay between mind and body has both an inward, subjective expression and an outward, objective expression.

The subjective expression is the experience of emotion. What we feel. The language we use to describe emotions reveals the connection between mind and body: "I feel." "I was hurt." "My heart was broken." "I was crushed." "My head was spinning." It seems that there are more physical references to negative emotions than positive emotions. There are more metaphors for negative emotions than positive. Emotions are associated with very measurable changes in the body, many of which produce physical sensations. These are well documented: The heart rate changes; blood flow is directed from one part of the body to the other; secretions in the digestive system are altered; sweat glands become more active. When we experience emotions we experience the inward expression of the mind-body interplay.

When experiencing emotions, we experience the most immediate evidence for the dynamic interplay between mind and body. Some would ascribe emotions as being "psychological," relegating this so very important part of our selves to "the mind." But this does not resonate with our real experience. Emotions, though certainly involving thoughts, are nearly always physical. Consider the very language we use to describe emotions: We "feel" emotions; "my heart is broken;" "my heart sank;" "my heart was pounding with excitement;" "I was trembling with fear." The list goes on. Emotions, nearly always experienced with physical sensations, and nearly always accompanied by certain thoughts, are the private expression of the mind-body connection.

The public or objective expression of the dynamic interplay between mind and body is *behavior*. Our thoughts and beliefs (mind), our physical selves, and our emotions always translate into behavior—what we do or do not do. To do anything at all is by definition physical (body), but on the most basic level it also involves a choice (mind). All behavior is a choice. Even behavior which we are forced to do is a choice: We could choose not to do a certain thin; we would just have to bear the consequences. The majority of health concerns in this country, the symptoms and conditions that interfere with quality and quantity of life—what it means to be healthy as we have defined that term—are directly related to our behavior. It follows, then, that if we are to soundly consider what it takes to be healthy, we must focus on behavior. But behavior does not occur in a vacuum: It is the observable, public product of the complex interactions between our thoughts and beliefs, our bodies, and our emotions: each affecting the other; each playing their role in our health.

Modern science supports this premise. Though it has long been known that medications, which alter the body's chemistry, can alter our experience of what we call the mind (our thoughts and perceptions), we now know from neuroscience that as human beings learn, new synapses, or connections between neurons in our brain, are formed. There is powerful scientific data to support the idea that the subjective experience of stress (self-perceptions made up of thoughts, emotions, and physical sensations) has profound effects on the immune system, the cardiovascular system, and the neuroendocrine system.

So it is imperative that as we consider *health*, we consider the self as a *whole* (recall the root word these terms share). I will argue (and I am by far not the first to do so) that it is very useful—indeed, very healthy—to consider the self as a dramatic interplay between our minds and our bodies; that this interplay finds its inward expression in our emotions and its outward expression in our behavior.

In a subsequent chapter, we will return in more detail to this concept of behavior and its link to thoughts, emotions, our bodies' performance, and achieving health.

CHAPTER 2
HEALTH AND DISEASE

The medical and public health community traditionally thinks of health in terms of a few categories. These categories capture the primary measures of health in terms of outcomes that can be analyzed and hopefully acted upon. They are:

1) Disease incidence: The number of new cases of a particular disease over a given amount of time.
2) Disease prevalence: The number of cases that exist at a given point or period of time.
3) Disease burden. The measurable consequences of disease. Typical measures of disease burden are mortality, morbidity, disability, and cost.

Incidence and prevalence can be tricky, and their measure is determined primarily by how common a condition or disease is and how long it lasts. Consider 100 business professionals sitting in a room. If we poll these people we will find the following:

1) About 75% of them will have had a headache in the last year. This would reflect incidence, or the number of new cases in the last year. The incidence is high because headache is a very common condition.
2) About 5% of them will have a headache *right now*. This reflects prevalence. The prevalence is low because headache, though very common, does not last very long, so the number of cases currently is low.
3) About 60% of them will be overweight at the present time (prevalence). The prevalence is high not only because being overweight is a common problem but also because it is a condition that typically lasts a long period of time.
4) Perhaps 2-3% of the group actually became overweight in the last year. The incidence is low because it takes years to become overweight, so the number of new cases is far fewer than the number of current cases.

These concepts are important because conditions that are chronic, or long-lasting, affect a cumulative burden to society, even if the number of new cases each year is relatively low. Conditions that are both common and long lasting confer, of course, an even greater burden.

So how is burden usually considered? In a few ways. The most rudimentary measure is mortality rate, usually expressed as the number of deaths per year. Next is morbidity, which refers to the consequences of disease other than mortality. These are more difficult to define and measure, and include pain, disability, days lost from work, and "quality of life" scores based on standardized questionnaires. Lastly, burden refers to the direct and indirect costs of a disease. Cost can refer to the personal costs to the person experiencing the disease or cost to society in general. Not surprisingly, the greater the disease's mortality and morbidity, the greater the cost.

Although in this book we are focusing primarily on your particular health, considering the above concepts will serve to frame our approach to living a healthy life, especially as we focus on the staggering burden that is wrought by unhealthy behavior.

CHAPTER 3
THE MIRACLE OF MODERN MEDICINE

Modern medicine considers disease and illness from two perspectives: prevention and treatment. Though we know a great deal about treatment of illness, we now know a great deal about preventing illness in the first place. Most Americans consider going to the doctor when they feel ill. Most primary care physicians would like people to consider going to the doctor when they feel well. Why? Because most of the disease burden in this country—defined as mortality, morbidity, and cost—is *preventable*. I repeat: Most of the disease burden in this country is preventable. If we consider mortality rates alone, *nearly half* the deaths in this country could be prevented *entirely by a change in behavior*. Not by pills or new tests, not even by the discovery of "culprit" genes, but by the public expression of the mind-body connection: by behavior. In addition, it is through behavior that you can achieve health—not only as defined by the absence of disease burden—but as defined by a thriving life. To thrive, not just survive. That is the goal. And it is attainable.

Modern medicine aims to prevent the onset of disease and to prevent or reduce the burden of that disease. To refer to these efforts, clinical epidemiology utilizes the concepts of *primary prevention* and *secondary prevention*. Primary prevention refers to prevention of illness in the first place, for example, preventing the onset of diabetes in someone not known to have that disorder already. Secondary prevention refers to efforts taken to prevent the consequences of a disease in someone already known to have the disorder. For example, preventing a heart attack in someone known to have coronary artery disease, or preventing another stroke in someone who has already suffered one. When considering the diseases and conditions responsible for the majority of disease burden in this country, treatment rarely means "cure." Most "treatments" are efforts at secondary prevention, in preventing the consequences of known illness. For example, there are specific, effective treatments for myocardial infarction or heart attacks, which are known to reduce the chances that a person will die from that event, but the person is still left with coronary artery disease, for which there is no cure.

From society's standpoint, and I believe an individual's standpoint, modern medicine offers much more in the way of disease prevention than in disease treatment. But what modern medicine offers is all too frequently ignored today, probably because it primarily offers sound advice: sound advice about behavior. This book is mainly about that good advice and what it takes to really hear it—to really take it to heart!

Treatment refers to interventions designed to reduce the burden of disease in those known to have that disease. Identifying those with disease is, of course, the first step to treatment. After sound advice about behavior, the most important thing modern medicine offers is the means to identify disease in the first place. A large number of simple tests and procedures are available today, which can identify people with the most common, chronic, and burdensome diseases. (We will discuss these in detail in a later chapter.) What's more, clinical epidemiology has given us the tools not only to identify those who already have a disease, but those *at risk* of getting the disease. That risk is in many cases measurable. It is also in most cases *changeable*. The primary vehicle of that change is, of course, behavior.

CHAPTER 4
TAKING A STATISTICAL APPROACH

Let us turn to a more statistical, epidemiological consideration of health and disease. We will start by considering disease burden. First, let's consider mortality, or the number of deaths per year. Table X provides data from the U.S. population for the year 2000. If we look at this list and consider just the chronic disease states, which include heart disease, stroke, cancer, chronic lung disease, and diabetes, we see that these diseases make up nearly 70% of all deaths in this country. That translates into more than 1.7 million American deaths each year. What about burden other than mortality? If we consider disability, we know from recent survey data that one in 10 Americans experiences a significant limitation in daily living because of these diseases. If we consider cost, we will find that caring for these conditions makes up nearly 75% of the 1 trillion dollars spent each year in this country on healthcare. These conditions, then, lead to 70% of the deaths, at least 10% of the disability, and nearly 75% of the health care expenditures in this country each year. These data are all the more staggering since so much of the toll exacted by these conditions is *preventable*.

How is it preventable? Not by modern technology, not by new medications, not by new diagnostic tests, or exciting new cures like gene therapy, but by *behavior*—what we do and what we do not do—what we choose to do and choose not to do.

There is an abundance of scientific data to support the premise that change in our population's behavior could lead to substantial increases in life expectancy, reductions in disability, and astounding health care cost savings. Table Y compares the leading causes of death based on *disease* to the *actual* causes of death, which, as can be seen plainly, are most likely to be behavior.

TABLE Y
Causes of Death in the United States

Most   **Common,**   **1999***

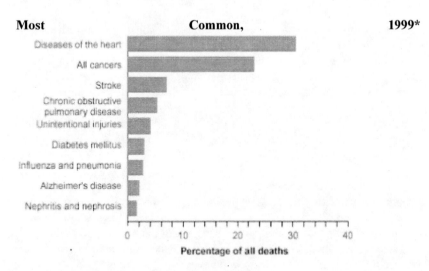

Actual,   **1990**   †

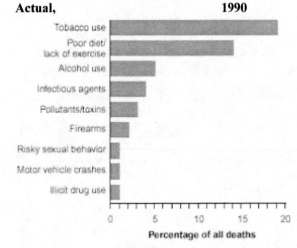

All data are age adjusted to 2000 total U.S. population.
† McGinnis JM, Foege WH. Actual causes of death in the United States.
JAMA 1993; 270:2207–12.

And that is if we consider health merely from the standpoint of mortality! Though reductions in mortality are a goal in medicine, if we continue to consider health as we have defined it---not by how many survive, but how many thrive—the benefits of healthy behavior are even more profound.

We will now focus on the relatively few conditions that contribute to the majority of disease burden in our country and examine them more closely.

Diabetes

The incidence and prevalence of diabetes is on the rise. If current trends continue, it is estimated that nearly 1 in 10 adults in this country will have diabetes by the year 2025! This chronic disease is the leading cause of blindness, amputation, and kidney failure in the United States. In addition, the risk of having heart disease for someone with diabetes is so high that the American Heart Association recommends diabetic patients be treated as "coronary artery disease equivalents." It is estimated that nearly a third of the 16 million Americans who have diabetes—or about 5 million people— do not even know they have the disease because it can be clinically silent for years!

Obesity

Much noise has been made in the popular media and medical literature regarding the "epidemic" of obesity—with good reason. The prevalence of obesity in this country has doubled since 1980. One in five Americans is now obese! (Mokdad, et al, JAMA 2003;289:76-79) The chart below provides a visual portrayal of this staggering increase in a condition that is nearly entirely rooted in behavior. In the next decade, obesity is expected to replace cigarette smoking as the *leading reversible cause of death* in the United States. A recent study estimated that adults who are obese at age 40 have a 6- to 7-year reduction in life-expectancy compared to similar adults who are not obese. If these obese adults smoke cigarettes, that loss of life-expectancy increases to 13 to 14 years! (Ann Intern Med.2003;138:24-32; Peeters, et al.)

Dr. Kevin Fosnocht

Percentage of Adults Who Report Being Obese,* by State

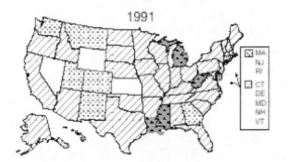

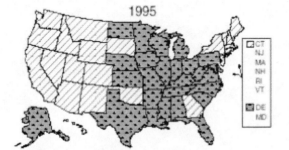

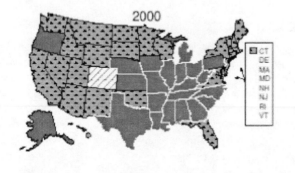

☐ No data available   ⊡ <10%   ▨ 10%–14%   ▦ 15%–19%   ■ ≥20%

*Body mass index greater than or equal to 30 or about 30 pounds overweight for a 5'4" person.
Source: CDC, Behavioral Risk Factor Surveillance System.

Cancer

Cancer is the second most common cause of death in the United States, accounting for almost one in every four deaths each year, which translates to over 500,000 cancer deaths a year. Though the term cancer applies to a multitude of illnesses, with complex genetic, environmental, and behavioral factors at work, it is estimated that about *one-third* of cancer deaths in this country are due to cigarette smoking alone. Another third are due to nutritional factors, physical inactivity, and obesity for a total of 60% *of cancer deaths attributable to behavior.* In addition, another kind of behavior—undergoing recommended screening and early detection examinations—can also substantially reduce the number of cancers and the number of cancer deaths.

Disability

We have just considered mortality rates as one measure of disease burden. The conditions that account for the majority of deaths in this country, especially heart disease and cancer, could be tremendously reduced in number with changes in behavior. But what about other measures of disease burden? If we move from causes of death and consider disability, we see a similar pattern. Disability in this context refers to loss of complete normal function and serves as a measure of the quality, as opposed to quantity, of life. Table A lists the most common causes of disability among adults in this country. It is no surprise that we see heart disease, lung disease, stroke and diabetes as substantial contributors to disability, these being chronic conditions and frequent causes of death in the United States. However, the leading causes of disability in this country are related to joint and back pain. It is estimated that one in six Americans suffers from arthritis or other rheumatic conditions. By 2020, it is predicted that that number will increase to include one in five Americans. Though most consider these conditions a problem of the elderly, the data do not support that assumption: Nearly three in five people with arthritis are *younger* than age 65!

Dr. Kevin Fosnocht

Most Common Causes of Disability Among Americans Aged 18 Years or Older, 1999

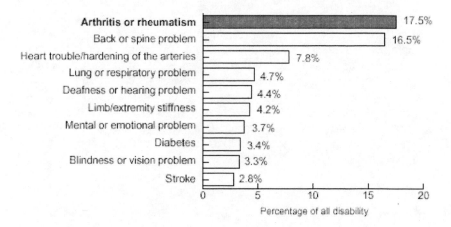

Source: CDC. Prevalence of disabilities and associated health conditions among adults —United States, 1999. MMWR2001; 50:120–5.

Estimated Arthritis Prevalence, 1990 and Projected to 2020

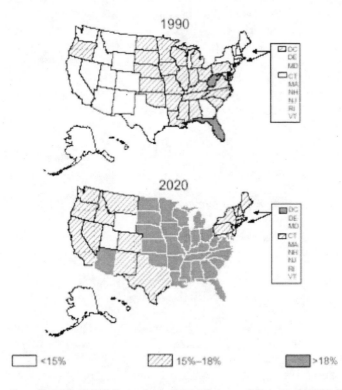

Source: Helmick CG, et al. Arthritis Care and Research 1995;8:203–11.

After joint pain, heart, lung and hearing problems, what is the next most common cause of disability? Mental or emotional problems. Public health studies show that up to 24% of adults in this country have experienced a mental disorder during the preceding year and an estimated 10% have some recent disability from a diagnosable mental illness. In a nationwide survey conducted from 1993 to 1996, nearly one in 10 adults said their mental health "was not good" for over 13 of the last 30 days. (BRFSS 1993-96; MMWR Weekly Report; May 1, 1998/ 47(16); 325331)

Depression is more common than most people realize—or at least more common than people are willing to acknowledge and talk about.

Approximately 18.8 million American adults, or about 9.5 % of the U.S. population age 18 and older in a given year have a depressive disorder. (NIMH) Somewhere between 5% and 10% of people seen in primary care settings—those who go to the doctor—meet criteria for major depression. Those criteria include at least two weeks of depressed mood or lack of enjoyment in things one used to enjoy *and* at least four of the following symptoms: fatigue, sleep problems, unintentional weight loss or gain, slow or agitated thinking, inability to concentrate, feelings of guilt, recurrent thoughts of death, etc. It is estimated that three times as many people have many of these depressive symptoms but do not meet the formal criteria described. We call this minor depression. Not surprisingly, both minor and major depression are associated with substantial disability. Depression is the fourth most important cause of disability worldwide.

Anxiety disorders are another common condition that have substantial effects on disability. Approximately 19.1 million American adults ages 18 to 54, or about 13.3 % of people in this age group in a given year have an anxiety disorder. (NIMH)

There is considerable overlap of depression and anxiety. Many patients have both and it is difficult to determine which is more operative in their lives.

Taken together, depression and anxiety are probably the most common diagnoses primary care physicians could make. But studies have shown that physicians miss the diagnosis about half the time. Though many of these cases are missed because the physician did not ask the right questions, many more are likely missed because patients who come to their doctors usually come with *physical complaints*, not complaints about mood. These complaints are real. They are not "psychological." If we consider our model of the whole person—in the context of the mind-body connection—it does not make sense to consider physical symptoms as "psychological." Depression and anxiety are disorders with physical symptoms. These symptoms vary greatly from patient to patient. They are a significant reason why so many business professionals, and people in general, feel as though they are just surviving—and far from thriving.

What happens if we combine mortality and disability and consider their cumulative effect on the quantity and quality of life? Epidemiologists are able to combine the statistics used to determine mortality and disability and express them in a single term: "disability-adjusted-life-year" or DALY. This term measures lost years of healthy life regardless of whether the years were lost to premature death or disability. The World Health Organization, the World Bank, and Harvard University combined efforts to conduct a world-wide study called the *Global Burden of Disease*. Among other things, this study determined the major causes of lost years of healthy life across the world expressed in disability-adjusted-life-years. Based on our review of causes of mortality and disability thus far, the results of this study were not surprising. The table below expresses the top 10 causes of DALYs for developed nations, including ours.

The Leading Sources of Disease Burden in Established Market Economies, 1990,

(measured in DALYs*)

		Total (millions)	Percent of Total
	All Causes	98.7	
1.	Ischemic heart disease	8.9	9.0
2.	**Unipolar major depression**	6.7	6.8
3.	Cardiovascular disease	5.0	5.0
4.	Alcohol use	4.7	4.7
5.	Road traffic accidents	4.3	4.4
6.	Lung & UR cancers	3.0	3.0
7.	Dementia & degenerative CNS	2.9	2.9
8.	Osteoarthritis	2.7	2.7
9.	Diabetes	2.4	2.4
10.	COPD	2.3	2.3

Global Burden of Disease Report, WHO/Harvard School of Public Health/World Bank; Summary of Global Burden of Disease; (ed., Murray, C; Lopez, A)

What is surprising in this list is not the conditions listed, but the rank of the conditions. Depression ranks as the second most common cause of loss of years of healthy life. If we combine depression, other mental illnesses, and alcohol abuse, we find that these conditions are responsible for more lost years of healthy life *than all cancers combined*. This kind of data gets more to the core of what we mean when we consider how best to thrive, not just survive. It is years of a *healthy* life, a *whole* life, indeed, (dare we go so far as to say?) a *holy* life that we want.

CHAPTER 5
WHAT MODERN MEDICINE OFFERS: ADVICE AND TECHNOLOGY

Centuries of observation, experience, and reflection eventually opened the door to the Scientific Revolution in the 16th century. Since then, humankind has achieved tremendous advances in understanding human anatomy and physiology and applied that knowledge to the pursuit of health. Much of that understanding has been achieved in the last 50 years, when technology allowed observation at the molecular and genetic level. This technology has spawned virtual miracles: antibiotics, vaccinations, general anesthesia, neurosurgery, cardiac bypass, life support systems, and organ transplant to name a few. Medicine offers all of this and much more.

But I propose that this technology, however important, offers little in comparison to what else medicine offers: advice. By "advice," I do not mean simply a few good suggestions that might "help," but rather data-driven facts whose value can be visibly measured by quantity and quality of life.

The most powerful advice, of course, is advice about our behavior—what to do or not to do—where to go. But one cannot give advice about direction until one first has a clear understanding of where one is at the moment. Modern medicine offers great insight into our health status—the "where we are" point. It relies on some basic measures afforded by science and technology as well as carefully studied observations about populations and illness (epidemiology). By combining the two (basic measures of our anatomy and physiology, and epidemiologic data), we can begin to understand our own health status then follow the advice medicine offers to achieve a healthy life.

Understanding Your Health in Terms of Risk

Epidemiologists use the term "risk" to describe the chances that some event will occur in a particular group. Usually expressed as a percentage, to refer to the number of people in the group that will experience the event, risk frequently refers to the chances of getting a disease or the chances of suffering the consequences of a disease. It is a prediction of sorts, based on years of study of prior observations. The most basic expression of risk in a population is simply the frequency of that event in the population over a given period of time. If that concept sounds identical to "incidence," it is! Incidence, or the number of new cases of some condition, when expressed as a percent of a group being studied, is the average risk that that condition will occur.

Epidemiology has discovered that there are certain identifiable factors that can increase or decrease the chances that you develop a certain condition. These are called "risk factors." We usually use the simple term "risk factor," to refer to positive risk factors or those risk factors that increase the chances that a condition develops. However, for many conditions there are "negative risk factors" that have been shown to decrease the chances that a condition develops.

Risk factors are considered to be either modifiable or nonmodifiable. Modifiable risk factors are attributes that can be changed through behavior, such as weight, cholesterol level, and blood pressure. Nonmodifiable risk factors are unchangeable attributes like age, sex, and a family history of a disorder.

Over the last few decades, modern epidemiology has made great strides in identifying risk factors for many of the important disorders discussed in the previous chapter. Doing so has allowed us to develop and target interventions, in the case of modifiable risk factors, and to determine who might be in need of a more aggressive assessment, in the case of nonmodifiable risk factors.

Clinical epidemiology and newer technologies have allowed us to quickly calculate the risk of acquiring some of the most common and burdensome diseases. In the Appendix are the web sites for accessing these easy to use, and readily explained, "risk calculators."

Self Assessment Tools (Appendix)

In the preceding chapters we have considered the concepts of disease burden and disease risk. These issues are extremely important as we embark on a pursuit of health. Assessing risk and hopefully modifying risk of disease are integral to maintaining health—at least from the standpoint of surviving. In later chapters, we will target reducing risk as a major goal of healthy living. But what about thriving? What about the quality of the life we lead? As we noted earlier, conditions such as arthritis and emotional orders actually contribute more disease burden world wide than does cancer! Every day in my medical practice I see patients whose illnesses, i.e., the very human experience of impaired health, is caused not merely by disease, but of the concern over symptoms generated by unhealthy behavior. Often their disease, if not caused by, is at least either exacerbated or complicated by, unhealthy behavior. It is often extremely difficult to tease out whether or not their symptoms find their origin in the disease process itself or in their behaviors.

In the first chapter we defined behavior as the outward expression, the public expression, of the mind-body interaction. We concluded that behavior is not merely a product of that interaction, but that behavior itself can affect our minds, certainly our bodies, and, consequently, our emotions, which are the internal expression of the mind-body interaction.

We outlined the degree to which behavior plays a role in the degree of disease burden. Not much of this is hot off the press news: Behavior has profound effects on health, perhaps more profound than genetics or the environment, especially in the 21st century, when we are so able to fight the larger scourges of earlier times, particularly infection, at least in developed countries.

But what behaviors lead to the most benefit? What behaviors can take us beyond merely surviving and lead to a truly thriving life? We will attempt to answer these questions, but the reader will not be surprised by the answers. What will be surprising is the degree to which these behaviors are not practiced and the utter lack of an apparent reason why they are not.

I would go so far as to say that *at least half* of the disease burden my patients suffer would simply (though not easily) disappear by making sustained, deliberate choices to do the following:

1) **Move**
2) **Eat well**
3) **Sleep well**
4) **Cultivate Meaning**
5) **Seek preventive care with your doctor**

These are not novel insights into healthy living. These are simple prescriptions. Accurate information on the "hows" and "whats" of these prescriptions is critical if one if to achieve the benefits I and others claim they afford, and I will provide that information. But several of the behaviors listed above quite easily pass the simple test of common sense. That is, through science, technology, public health efforts, and the media most people today recognize that exercise and diet, for example, are critical to maintaining health. They might not know the degree to which these behaviors can improve health, or exactly what kinds of exercise or what kinds of food are the most beneficial, but most people know that exercising and eating right are good for you.

Yet in 2003 we find that the U.S. population as a whole is the most sedentary and overweight that it has ever been! Obesity, diabetes, arthritis, and depression are on the rise! Why are so many people not heeding this simple advice? Why are so many not hearing the message and in fact doing the opposite? Why do the majority of people in this country not take the simple steps listed above? What is—what are the barriers?

I do not accept the argument that our society is simply lazy and gluttonous. We as a country have achieved far too much in every aspect of life over the last century to chalk the epidemics of obesity and diabetes up to mere laziness. In fact, as I talk to my patients, I find that the barriers they encounter to regularly practicing healthy behaviors have little to do with laziness. They are achieving near Herculean goals professionally and in their family lives. They are often exhausted by the degree of work that goes in to maintaining these aspects of their lives. No, it is not laziness. Most Americans work too hard to say it is laziness. Let's consider the healthy behaviors of diet and exercise. If we know the benefits (mind), are able to physically practice the behavior (body), and feel guilty or shameful that we don't (emotions), why are we not achieving the behavior?

To answer this question, it is necessary to return to our discussion of the relationship between the mind and body. If behavior is the outward or public expression of the mind-body interaction, and if emotions are its inward expression, and if emotions themselves affect the mind and body, then it is quite consistent to posit that these emotions also affect behavior. Our minds (thoughts, beliefs, personality traits), our emotions (feelings and their physical sensations), and our bodies (both predetermined genetic aspects and consequences of our environment), are all involved in our behavior. More simply put, every behavior is associated with a thought and an emotion. Moreover, every behavior is, ultimately, a choice. It follows, then, that if we are to make deliberate, sustainable choices to live healthy lives—in particular, to practice healthy behavior— then we must, in an ongoing process, carefully consider the thoughts and emotions that accompany our behavior, be it healthy or unhealthy.

How can this kind of careful consideration be achieved? I will argue that making deliberate, sustainable choices to live healthy lives—to thrive, not just survive—includes and is absolutely dependent on some kind of structured, critical, self-reflection. In a word: psychotherapy—and I use the word deliberately in an attempt to demystify and clarify its meaning.

Psychotherapy refers to a variety of techniques employed by trained psychologists, psychiatrists, and other therapists, which usually involve dialogue as the primary means of treatment. There are many different types of psychotherapy, each based on a variety of particular assumptions about how people think, learn, cope with difficult situations, and behave. What they have in common is deliberate, guided reflection on one's thoughts and beliefs, emotions, and behaviors, with the goal of altering at least one of those to improve health.

Many people think of psychotherapy as reserved for those with severe mental illness, such as schizophrenia. Others would think it is reserved for those with an obviously psychological or emotional problem, such as substance abuse, severe depression, suicide attempts, or problems related to a history of some trauma, such as sexual abuse or bereavement. Psychotherapy certainly is a primary and effective means of treatment in all these situations, but does it have a role in the absence of these situations?

I would argue that it does. I think that most of us, to varying degrees, have barriers to achieving the kind of thriving life we desire. We have roadblocks, many self-constructed, which impede our ability to make deliberate, sustained choices to practice healthy behavior, particularly the healthy behavior components I have outlined and will discuss in detail in the remainder of this book.

Most of us go through our lives with our X locked in replay. The dynamic interplay between our thoughts, emotions, our bodies and behaviors moves—but it moves in set patterns for a given set of circumstances.

To illustrate how these patterns play a role in our lives, consider the following situation:

You are driving in your car to a meeting. You are not late but have allotted yourself "just enough" time. You come upon a traffic accident, a minor fender bender that has traffic at a standstill. You have to wait until the accident clears, as there is no way you can move your car out of its current position. These are the facts. Let's consider the thoughts, emotions, and behaviors that are the result of these facts.

Thoughts	Emotions	Behavior
"I should have never come this way. There's always a traffic jam!"	Guilt Self-reproach Frustration	Make attempts to move your car, even though it is not possible.
"I didn't expect this. It looks like I'll be late. Some things just can't be predicted."	Regret Resignation Neutral	Phone the person you're meeting and explain the situation.
"No one can drive in this town! If people would just use their heads, we'd all get to where we need to go."	Anger	Honk your horn.

We have all been in this situation, and very likely we have all experienced, at different times, each of the thought/emotion/behavior clusters described above. Modern psychology, however, tells us that our reactions to events like the one just described and, more importantly, to events that are much more serious, such as an illness, are fairly consistent across time and in varied situations. We have learned these responses, and we practice them daily. Most of us have a very large catalogue of thought/emotion/behavior clusters that we repeat without realizing it. I believe this offers an explanation for why we as a society are literally able to acknowledge one thing, but feel "compelled" to do another; why we know that obesity is an enormous health risk, but we are getting fatter; why we know that exercise affords enormous health benefits, but we are becoming more sedentary. Psychotherapy is designed to put a spotlight on these patterns and use proven techniques to change them to promote a healthier, fuller life.

Several years ago, a business executive in his mid-40s came to me for primary care upon referral from a cardiologist. He had originally seen the cardiologist because his father had died of a heart attack a few years earlier, and he wanted to get "checked out." In fact, his overall health was quite good: He did not have high blood pressure or diabetes; he did not smoke; and though he had high cholesterol, this was being treated successfully with medication. He was, however, quite sedentary, getting basically no leisure time physical activity. He related to me that he found his being sedentary quite odd, since he had been a regular runner and athlete throughout his youth and into college. He also told me that he had frequent bouts of insomnia, especially over the last year or so, and explained it by "all the stress of the day." I told him that if he was really interested in reducing his risk of a heart attack and improving his sleep, he would get regular, vigorous exercise. He agreed—and went on his way.

I saw him in follow-up a few months later. He had gained a couple of pounds, and no, he had not found the time to exercise. I decided to take a different approach than offering "tips" on the benefits of exercise. I explained to him that his not exercising was a behavior, and that this behavior was very likely to be locked in a pattern with certain thoughts and feelings. Maybe the clue to his behavior was in considering these thoughts and feelings. I asked him a simple question: "When you consider exercising or exerting yourself how do you feel?" He paused for a moment to reflect. He seemed a bit ill at ease, so I probed further: "You seem a little distressed by my question. Am I right?" "Yes", he replied. "Then tell me what you are thinking right now," I instructed. He said, "I'm thinking of my father." "Your father", I reflected, though I was somewhat surprised. He became visibly more distressed. I asked again, "What are your feelings right now?" "To tell you the truth, Doctor, I'm really scared. I'm really scared of having a heart attack and dying." He then went on to describe how when he exerted himself and felt his heart beat, he was worried that he would die. He knew this thought to be somewhat irrational, but the thoughts led to emotions that he tried to avoid. So he couldn't bring himself to exercise because of the thoughts and feelings associated with his father's death and the potential risk it meant to him. He then related that it was this same thought and emotion cycle that kept him up at night and which he found very difficult to stop.

I referred him to a psychotherapist colleague of mine, so that he could work through these thoughts and emotions with the goal of changing his behavior. Within several months he was exercising regularly and sleeping better. He was so impressed with the psychologist that he brought the psychologist into his business to address important employee interactions.

This anecdote illustrates the importance of critical self-reflection if we are to change our behavior to live a thriving life. With this in mind, let me make some intentionally provocative claims. If you are 30 lbs overweight and have knee arthritis that causes daily pain, you need psychotherapy. If you smoke and "can't quit," you need psychotherapy. If you are fatigued, and your physician has told you that all the tests "are normal," and you do not exercise, you need therapy. I would argue that if you are overweight, do not exercise, sleep poorly, or don't go to a doctor for regular check-ups, you need therapy. You do not necessarily (though you might) need the type and/or duration of therapy used to treat severe depression, but you need some kind of guided critical reflection if you want to make deliberate, sustained choices to practice healthy behavior. I feel confident about these claims because if you did not need guided, critical reflection in your life, you would, naturally, be pursuing healthy living. You would want to take simple, low risk, ultimately enjoyable steps to not just survive, but to thrive. This argument is nothing more than Socrates' adage that "the unexamined life is not worth living." Therapy is nothing less than examining your life.

Why do we need to involve someone else, a therapist, a "total stranger?" Why can't we simply promise ourselves we will carefully consider our thoughts, emotions, and behavior and change them to live healthier lives? For a couple of reasons. First, critical reflection takes effort and know-how. There are proven techniques which can more efficiently and accurately help us to critically appraise our behavior. The second reason is a bit more philosophical. Someone once said "we only know as much about ourselves as we are willing to admit to others." There is something important about sharing our impressions with another human being: getting an objective assessment of our own thoughts and emotions. This kind of sharing leads to self-knowledge. Therapists are trained to remain objective and not let us deceive ourselves about what we are truly thinking, feeling, and, for that matter, doing.

Martin Seligman, PhD, a well-known psychologist at the University of Pennsylvania, has theorized that individuals explain or experience events that occur in their lives from three different angles. (1) We ascribe a "cause" of an event as being "internal" or "external," i.e., the cause is generated by our own doing or is beyond our reach, outside of our control. (2) We believe the cause of the event is "stable" or "unstable," meaning a particular event is predictable or "always" happens, or is random and things could certainly have happened differently. (3) We believe events are "global" or "specific," meaning "things like this always happen" or that the events are particular to this situation, time, and place.

Think about the trivial event of the traffic jam described above. Here is an example of an internal/stable/global explanation of the events:

"I should never have come this way (internal). There is always a traffic jam here (stable). Things like this always happen to me (global)."

An external/unstable/specific explanation would sound like this:

"Looks like an accident up ahead. Someone was probably not paying attention (external). I haven't seen an accident here in a few months (unstable). Looks like I'll be late for my meeting. If we had decided to meet an hour earlier we might have not run into this mess (specific)."

Seligman's research suggests that the "explanatory style" that we have is mostly learned and applied consistently to explain or make sense of events in our lives. The businessman who explains events in an internal/stable/global way tends to be pessimistic. The businessman who explains events in an external/unstable/specific way is optimistic. When researchers identify people who have a pessimistic explanatory style, they are found, not surprisingly, to have higher rates of clinical depression than those who have optimistic explanatory styles. What is more, Seligman's research strongly suggests that those who are optimistic are *healthier*. His research has also shown that optimism (like pessimism) can be learned. (See more about this study in chapter W.)

So, does everyone need therapy? In a word, yes. I do not claim that everyone needs long-standing, intense therapy, but I do believe that to truly thrive, one needs to engage in critical self-reflection—and that is best done through someone trained in techniques that facilitate that kind of reflection. Put another way, if you cannot seriously engage in the healthy behaviors outlined in this book on a regular basis, you should have some kind of therapy, at some time, for some duration. Psychotherapy can teach what the American Psychological Association calls *resilience*, which is characterized by the capacity to manage strong feelings and impulses, skill in communication and problem solving, confidence in your strengths and abilities, and, perhaps most importantly relative to the purpose of this book, the capacity to make realistic plans and take steps to carry them out. (*The Road to Resilience*, American Pyschological Association Practice directorate)

CHAPTER 6
TAKING THE STEPS: SIMPLE BUT NOT EASY

The steps to healthy living are by no means revolutionary. They are simple. They are so basic, in fact, that it is difficult to find an argument that would impugn any one of them. Not only is there ample scientific data to suggest they are important to both surviving and thriving, they also pass the test of common sense. One cannot be healthy—as we have defined that term—without exercise, nutrition, rest, and active participation in the interconnectedness of human beings. These steps are so simple that we as a society may have dismissed them as too simple.

Though simple, these steps are not easy. If they were both simple and easy, the problems of increasing rates of obesity, diabetes, depression, stress, sleep disturbance, arthritis, and cancer would not exist.

There is no lack of interest—or even money—on the part of the general population in matters of healthy living. According to a Harris Interactive poll, in 2000 an estimated 100 million consumers sought health information on the Internet (The Wall Street Journal, 12/29/00). In 1997, there were 629 million visits to practitioners of complementary and alternative medicine providers, a number exceeding the number of visits to primary care providers. The estimated out-of pocket expenditures that year on these visits and herbal remedies exceeded $30 billion! (Eisenberg DM, Davis RB, Ettner SI, et al. Trends in alternative medicine use in the United States, 1990-1997: results of a follow-up national survey. *JAMA*. 1998;280:1569-1575.) My own clinical practice supplies ample evidence to me in this regard. On a daily basis, I see patients who are not exercising, not eating well, and who have poor insight into the thoughts and emotions that accompany their behavior, yet have multiple questions about herbal remedies and are often spending large amounts of money on well-marketed "natural" supplements.

Before we describe the healthy behaviors in detail, it must be emphasized these are not meant to be temporary interventions. They must be steps taken quite regularly, if not daily, if one is to achieve the measurable, real benefits. These steps are based on sound science and clinical experience. But the responsibility is yours. You have to take the steps. You have to find a way to make deliberate, sustained choices to practice the healthy behaviors.

CHAPTER 7
PHYSICAL ACTIVITY IS THE KEY

After regular critical self-reflection, the most important healthy behavior is exercise. I will go so far as to say that if you do not engage in regular physical activity (and we will define that term) you are not and cannot be healthy. You might be surviving, but you are not thriving; and if you believe yourself to be thriving, yet are sedentary, not only do you not know what you are missing, you have a considerably higher risk of developing serious disease.

Historically, the physical labor inherent in day-to-day living and many kinds of jobs required physical activity. As we are ever more reliant on conveniences for work and travel, this kind of physical activity has diminished markedly. Getting regular physical activity today, more than ever before, requires deliberate, sustained choices.

Everyday in my medical practice I prescribe exercise to nearly all of my patients. Few are able to make regular physical activity a part of their lives. Though some of my patients respond to my advice with excuses like a hectic schedule, time pressures, physical complaints that might make exercise unpleasant, etc., I am always surprised by how *few* excuses I hear. Most of my patients readily appreciate the known benefits of exercise, say they have a desire to do so, but respond with a self-defeated "I know, Doctor, but I just can't seem to do it." There is a resignation in their voice, a self-deprecating, frustrated tone. There is guilt and denial. It seems so simple. It is simple. But it is not easy. Why is it not easy? Because it requires a change in *behavior*. We are locked—locked into behavior patterns that are the expression of the reciprocal determinism of our thoughts and emotions. Making and taking the time, consciously engaging in activity that has so many measurable benefits, takes deliberate, sustained choices. If you are not already doing it, if you "can't" exercise, then you are in need of critical self-reflection. You need psychotherapy, the first building block.

Before we review in detail the benefits of regular physical activity, let's consider what exactly regular physical activity means. The Centers for Disease Control and Prevention and the Office of the Surgeon General, define it as moderate activity at least five days a week.

What is moderate activity? It depends. The amount of energy you spend in an activity is dependent on the kind of activity, how long you do it, and how frequently you do it. One very useful definition is activity of such intensity that it would be a bit difficult to have a conversation. Thirty minutes of an activity of such intensity would qualify as moderate activity. The Table below offers some examples of moderate activity, ranging from less to more vigorous.

TABLE ZZ

Examples of moderate amounts of physical activity

Common Chores	Sporting Activities
Washing and waxing a car for 45-60 minutes	Playing volleyball for 45-60 minutes
Washing windows or floors for 45-60 minutes	Playing touch football for 45 minutes
Gardening for 30-45 minutes	Walking 13/4 miles in 35 minute (20min/mile)
Wheeling self in wheelchair 30-40 minutes	Basketball (shooting baskets) 30 minutes
Pushing a stroller 11/2 miles in 30 minutes	Bicycling 5 miles in 30 minutes
Raking leaves for 30 minutes	Dancing fast (social) for 30 minutes
Walking 2 miles in 30 minutes (15min/mile)	Water aerobics for 30 minutes
Shoveling snow for 15 minutes	Swimming Laps for 20 minutes
Stairwalking for 15 minutes	Basketball (playing game) for 15-20 minutes
	Bicycling 4 miles in 15 minutes
	Jumping rope for 15 minutes
	Running 11/2 miles in 15 min. (10min/mile)

Source: NHLBI: The Practical Guide for the Identification, Evaluation, and Treatment of Overweight and Obesity in Adults NIH Publication Number 00-4084; October 2000

Living Longer Working Stronger

A more specific and scientific definition of moderate activity is 30 minutes of activity that gets your heart beating to 60-80% of your maximum predicted heart rate (MPHR). There are many biological and physiological factors that go in to determining one's MPHR, but a functional and relatively accurate estimation can be determined by the following equation: MPHR (beats per minute) = 220-age (years). So if you are 50 years of age, your MPHR is (220-50) =170. 60-80% of that number is 102-136 beats per minute. You can determine your heart rate at any time by feeling your radial pulse (see figure) and counting the number of "beats" for 30 seconds, and multiplying that number by 2.

So how is America doing? Not very well. (See figure below) About 84% of Americans in 2000 were not getting the recommended amount of physical activity. Over one-quarter of Americans reported no physical activity! That number increases to about 30% if we include only people over 65 years of age and over 50% for people over 75.

What is the impact of this national sedentary status? Consider the following: a 1986 study published in JAMA suggested that 23% of deaths from the major chronic diseases were linked to the sedentary lifestyle. Given that the numbers who report being sedentary are even higher today, approximately 88 million Americans over the age of 15 years, we can assume that so too is the death toll from inactivity. A study performed by researchers at the CDC and published in 2000 estimated that increasing regular moderate physical activity among these inactive Americans could reduce annual national direct medical costs by as much as $76.6 billion! These are staggering data.

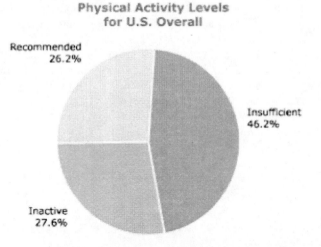

Physical Activity Levels
for U.S. Overall

Recommended 26.2%

Insufficient 46.2%

Inactive 27.6%

1. *Source:* **Behavioral Risk Factor Surveillance System 2000 (BRFSS).**
2. Data are weighted to each year's U.S. and state population estimates and age-adjusted to the year 2000 U.S. population standard.
3. Recommended = reported physical activity at least 5 times/week x 30 minutes/time or vigorous[6] physical activity for at least 20 minutes at a time at least 3 times/week.
4. Insufficient = any activity or pair of activities less than 5 times/week and 30 minutes/time and vigorous activity less than 3 times/week and 20 minutes/time.
5. Inactive = no reported physical activity.

I stated earlier that modern medicine offers advice and technology. The technologies that have advanced the health status of our country typically take the form of pills, shots, and procedures. None of these technologies, save perhaps vaccines, can be applied to nearly all ages, races, or both sexes. None can lead to improvement in nearly all organ systems simultaneously. None are without very measurable risks. Few are of low cost. Regular physical activity—exercise—can do all of these.

The word *exercise* comes from the Latin *exercere*, which literally means "to remove restraint." I enjoy this meaning of the word, because it conveys the principles of the building blocks to healthy living. Prior to engaging in healthy behavior, we must first remove the restraints that we, however unconsciously, have constructed around ourselves. We must critically reflect on the reciprocal determinism of our thoughts, emotions, and behaviors to make deliberate, sustained, choices.

Exercise is near the bottom of the building blocks of healthy living because it has the potential to sustain those above it. Exercise alters metabolism and the caloric balance necessary for weight loss and weight loss maintenance. It improves the quantity and quality of sleep. Regular physical activity is associated with less anxiety, improved mood, less tension, reduced stress, and an increased sense of overall well-being. These benefits are necessary to maintain the resilience to engage in the cultivation of relationships and the commitment to cultivate a spiritual life.

Let's consider for a moment what years of science have helped us conclude regarding the health benefits of regular physical activity.

Exercise can reduce the risk of developing or significantly improve the following disorders:

Cardiovascular disease
Diabetes
High blood pressure
Colon cancer
Obesity
Osteoarthritis
Depression
Osteoporosis

Does this list look familiar? It should. Most of these conditions are the leading causes of disease burden in our country. Let's more closely consider the effects of exercise on two of the main conditions which are dramatically affected by exercise, cardiovascular disease and diabetes.

In the last ·10 years, many large studies have examined the association between physical activity and risk of either developing or dying from coronary heart disease. The evidence suggests that there is a strong "dose-response" effect between exercise and risk of coronary heart disease. That means that the more activity you get on a regular basis (the dose), the less risk you have (response). People who are physically active, who undertake moderate levels of activity daily, can expect a *50% reduction* in risk of coronary heart disease, compared to those who are sedentary. Despite the successes of technology and the astounding advances in pharmaceutical development in the last 20 years, both of which have contributed substantially to the decreased mortality rates in coronary heart disease, *there is not a single intervention as efficacious as exercise in preventing coronary heart disease.* Technology—or advice? This is simply good advice.

What about exercise and stroke, the 3rd leading cause of death in this country? Again, the data have profound implications. Sedentary adults *are nearly twice as likely* to have a stroke than those who are moderately active. (Gillum RF, Mussolino ME, Ingram DD. Physical activity and stroke incidence in women and men: the NHANES I Epidemiologic Follow-up Study. *Am J Epidemiol.* 1996;143:860–869.) A recent study in New York City compared active to inactive older adults. The active adults participated in light to moderate activity, like that described in Table ZZ, for a total of about two hours during the week. The researchers found that the chances of stroke to be about 60% less in the active group, compared to their sedentary counterparts. The "dose-response" effect was seen in this study as well: People who engaged in vigorous activity for about 45 minutes a day were up to 75% less likely to have a stroke. (Sacco RL, Gan R, Boden-Albala B, et al. Leisure-time physical activity and ischemic stroke risk: the Northern Manhattan Stroke Study. *Stroke.* 1998;29:380–387.)

Let's consider diabetes. About 15% of the population, owing to the high rates of obesity and sedentary lifestyles, are at risk for developing diabetes. Two recently conducted, large, well-designed studies concluded that daily moderate activity, along with dietary counseling resulted in nearly a *60% reduction* in the development of diabetes. Again, no technological advance is as effective as behavioral change.

The evidence is quite clear and, in my opinion, quite inspiring! You do not need to be a marathon runner, a jogger, or a swimmer—you do not need to be an athlete at all, to get enormous benefits in reducing your risk of developing the leading causes of disease burden in this country. Though studies demonstrate that the more one exercises the more one achieves *fitness*, that is, strength and endurance for prolonged or difficult physical activity, the major health benefits, as we have just outlined, can be achieved with moderate activity. Fitness per se is a worthy goal and, in my opinion, provides enormous benefits. Again, no known technological therapy--- almost all of which have substantial risks and costs—is as comprehensively beneficial as regular physical activity. What you must do is move—and move daily.

Living Longer Working Stronger

The vast majority of studies that have documented the considerable health benefits of exercise have mostly examined the benefits of aerobic training, like walking, jogging, and biking. There are also very measurable benefits to resistance training and the American Heart Association recommends resistance exercise along with aerobic exercise to achieve the maximum benefit of regular physical activity. It appears that the health benefit—a reduction in the risk of diabetes, hypertension, coronary artery disease, and osteoporosis afforded by regular physical activity as we have defined it—can be augmented by resistance exercise. Ideally, this exercise regimen should include the following:

One or two sets of 10-15 repetitions of eight different exercises at least two days a week:

Chest press
Shoulder press
Triceps extension
Biceps curl
Pull-down bar
Abdominal crunch
Quadriceps extension or leg press
Leg curls (hamstrings)
Calf raise

Resistance exercise is especially important in weight management and in the prevention of diabetes. As we will discuss in the next chapter, the amount of lean body mass you have significantly determines your body's metabolism. Muscle is lean body mass. As you build muscle you enhance your body's ability to handle calories efficiently. This efficiency is necessary for optimal weight maintenance.

This kind of exercise also improves strength, of course, and has been shown to slow the age-related loss of bone mass which can lead to osteoporosis. In older people, resistance training has been shown to decrease the likelihood of falls. The strength developed from resistance training can add to feelings of self-confidence and enhance your overall sense of well-being.

In the box, then, are the official recommendations of the American Heart Association, adapted from its Guide to Primary Prevention of Cardiovascular Disease and Stroke: Risk Intervention.

GOAL: At least 30 minutes of moderate-intensity physical activity on most (and preferably all) days of the week. This 30-minute daily minimum can be achieved in a single 30 minute session, two 15-minute sessions, or three 10-minute sessions. Moderate-intensity activities are equivalent to a brisk walk (15-20 min per mile). Additional benefits are gained from vigorous-intensity activity for 20-40 min on 3-5d/week. Resistance training with 8-10 different exercises, 1-2 sets per exercise, and 10-15 repetitions at moderate intensity >/= 2d/wk.

(Pearson TA, Blair SN, et al., AHA Guidelines for Primary Prevention of Cardiovascular Disease and Stroke: 2002 Update. *Circulation*. 2002; 106:388-391.)

A note *for those who are currently sedentary* and considering taking the healthy step of increasing physical activity: If you are over 40 years of age or have any known cardiovascular (e.g., hypertension, coronary artery disease, blocked arteries), endocrine (e.g., diabetes, osteoporosis), respiratory (e.g., emphysema, chronic bronchitis), orthopedic (e.g., severe hip arthritis), or neurologic (e.g., spinal stenosis, history of stroke) disorder, consult a physician before beginning any exercise program. The risk of a cardiovascular or other problem with moderate activity is low, but if you already have known disease that risk may be higher. This word of caution especially applies to the very obese and to diabetics.

Starting Out

Many people, both in the business world and beyond, make resolutions to "get in shape," only to fail miserably. Health clubs, fitness centers, spas, and other types of membership-oriented exercise facilities make enormous profits because they know that people stop coming. Many a treadmill in many a home are used as very overpriced coat racks.

Health clubs and exercise equipment manufacturers have successfully sold the idea of fitness. They have been able to get the American public to spend millions each year in pursuit of this idea. Yet we are still left with the paradox that with each decade our population has become more sedentary, despite the enormous interest and expenditures on fitness.

If you are currently sedentary, start slowly. If you push yourself too hard too early, you will either get hurt or feel miserable and not be able to consider regular physical activity as a permanent and sustained life choice. Your ultimate goal should be to accumulate 30 minutes of moderate activity daily, but you will likely need to work up to that amount. So set initial goals that are both specific and realistic. Saying, "I'm going to exercise more every day" is neither specific nor realistic, especially for someone starting out. Saying, "I'm going to walk briskly for 10 minutes three days a week" is quite specific and very realistic. It will then be much easier to mark your success and work toward that ultimate goal of regular physical activity. Begin by daily walking, even if that walking is only for 10 minutes each day.

What follows are sample walking program and jogging programs published by the National Heart Lung and Blood Institute:

Dr. Kevin Fosnocht

A sample walking program

	Warmup	Exercising	Cool down	Total time
Week 1				
Session A	Walk 5 min.	Then walk briskly 5 min.	Then walk more slowly 5 min.	15 min.
Session B	Repeat above pattern			
Session C	Repeat above pattern			

Continue with at least three exercise sessions during each week of the program.

Week 2	Walk 5 min.	Walk briskly 7 min.	Walk 5 min.	17 min.
Week 3	Walk 5 min.	Walk briskly 9 min.	Walk 5 min.	19 min.
Week 4	Walk 5 min.	Walk briskly 11 min.	Walk 5 min.	21 min.
Week 5	Walk 5 min.	Walk briskly 13 min.	Walk 5 min.	23 min.
Week 6	Walk 5 min.	Walk briskly 15 min.	Walk 5 min.	25 min.
Week 7	Walk 5 min.	Walk briskly 18 min.	Walk 5 min.	28 min.
Week 8	Walk 5 min.	Walk briskly 20 min.	Walk 5 min.	30 min.
Week 9	Walk 5 min.	Walk briskly 23 min.	Walk 5 min.	33 min.
Week 10	Walk 5 min.	Walk briskly 26 min.	Walk 5 min.	36 min.
Week 11	Walk 5 min.	Walk briskly 28 min.	Walk 5 min.	38 min.
Week 12	Walk 5 min.	Walk briskly 30 min.	Walk 5 min.	40 min.

Week 13 on:

Gradually increase your brisk walking time to 30 to 60 minutes, three or four times a week. Remember that your goal is to get the benefits you are seeking and enjoy your activity.

Walking Tips

- Hold your head up, and keep your back straight.
- Bend your elbows as you swing your arms.
- Take long, easy strides.

For additional information about physical activity, request the NHLBI booklet *Exercise and Your Heart: A Guide to Physical Activity.*

Living Longer Working Stronger

A sample jogging program

If you are older than 40 and have not been active, you should not begin with a program as strenuous as jogging. Begin with the walking program instead. After completing the walking program, you can start with week 3 of the jogging program below.

	Warmup	Exercising	Cool down	Total time
Week 1				
Session A	Walk 5 min., then stretch and limber up	Then walk 10 min. Try not to stop.	Then walk more slowly 3 min. and stretch 2 min.	20 min.
Session B	Repeat above pattern			
Session C	Repeat above pattern			

Continue with at least three exercise sessions during each week of the program.

	Warmup	Exercising	Cool down	Total time
Week 2	Walk 5 min., then stretch and limber up	Walk 5 min., jog 1 min., walk 5 min., jog 1 min.	Walk 3 min., stretch 2 min.	22 min.
Week 3	Walk 5 min., then stretch and limber up	Walk 5 min., jog 3 min., walk 5 min., jog 3 min.	Walk 3 min., stretch 2 min.	26 min.
Week 4	Walk 5 min., then stretch and limber up	Walk 4 min., jog 5 min., walk 4 min., jog 5 min.	Walk 3 min., stretch 2 min.	28 min.
Week 5	Walk 5 min., then stretch and limber up	Walk 4 min., jog 5 min., walk 4 min., jog 5 min.	Walk 3 min., stretch 2 min.	28 min.
Week 6	Walk 5 min., then stretch and limber up	Walk 4 min., jog 6 min., walk 4 min., jog 6 min.	Walk 3 min., stretch 2 min.	30 min.
Week 7	Walk 5 min., then stretch and limber up	Walk 4 min., jog 7 min., walk 4 min., jog 7 min.	Walk 3 min., stretch 2 min.	32 min.
Week 8	Walk 5 min., then stretch and limber up	Walk 4 min., jog 8 min., walk 4 min., jog 8 min.	Walk 3 min., stretch 2 min.	34 min.
Week 9	Walk 5 min., then stretch and limber up	Walk 4 min., jog 9 min., walk 4 min., jog 9 min.	Walk 3 min., stretch 2 min.	36 min.
Week 10	Walk 5 min., then stretch and limber up	Walk 4 min., jog 13 min.	Walk 3 min., stretch 2 min.	27 min.
Week 11	Walk 5 min., then stretch and limber up	Walk 4 min., jog 15 min.	Walk 3 min., stretch 2 min.	29 min.
Week 12	Walk 5 min., then stretch and limber up	Walk 4 min., jog 17 min.	Walk 3 min., stretch 2 min.	31 min.
Week 13	Walk 5 min., then stretch and limber up	Walk 2 min., jog slowly 2 min., jog 17 min.	Walk 3 min., stretch 2 min.	31 min.
Week 14	Walk 5 min., then stretch and limber up	Walk 1 min., jog slowly 3 min., jog 17 min.	Walk 3 min., stretch 2 min.	31 min.
Week 15	Walk 5 min., then stretch and limber up	Jog slowly 3 min., jog 17 min.	Walk 3 min., stretch 2 min.	30 min.

Week 16 on: Gradually increase your jogging time from 20 to 30 minutes (or more, up to 60 minutes), three or four times a week. Remember that your goal is to get the benefits you are seeking and enjoy your activity.

Source: NHBLI

If you can accomplish this small amount of activity for a week or two, increase your walks to either two times daily or 20 minutes daily. If you can achieve that amount of activity for a few weeks you are ready to begin measuring your heart rate and aiming for 30 minutes of activity every day at a heart rate of 60-70% of your maximum. After several weeks of that level of activity, try to reach 70-80% of your maximum. You need not stick to walking. Table ZZ provides many examples of moderate activity. Varying the kinds of activities you do to achieve your goal will be more practical and certainly more enjoyable.

Many of my patients say that they do not have time to exercise. It is true, regular physical activity does take time. But as we have defined it, enormous health benefits can be achieved by as little as two hours spread out over a week's time. Considering that the average American watches *over three hours of television a day*, the time to exercise is certainly there. In my experience, people simply feel they don't have the time because, when the day's activities are near an end, they feel stressed and fatigued, overwhelmed with the daily activities of life. They are locked in a behavior pattern borne of the reciprocal determinism of their thoughts and emotions. That pattern includes having the behavior of television watching be a source of relaxation, stress reduction, and enjoyment. That pattern will lead to the average 65-year-old in this country having spent *nine years of life* watching television! Instituting behavior change that literally takes you off the couch and into the street requires a great deal of critical reflection. Can you really not find two 15-minute periods of time during the day to walk briskly? Or do you feel you can't find that time?

Reducing sedentary time, especially time spent watching television, is one of the most important strategies for successfully achieving regular physical activity. If you, for now, *must* watch television in the evenings, get on an exercise bicycle or use hand weights to achieve your activity goals while watching television.

Fatigue is a common symptom in my primary care practice. Fatigue is different from feeling sleepy. Most people can make the distinction between the two. Fatigue is a sense of not having energy to start or complete things that require physical, emotional, or mental exertion. Sleepiness just means that you feel the need to sleep. Most people with fatigue get plenty of sleep, but they are experiencing a lack of energy. Once my evaluation has ruled out a medical illness as the cause of fatigue, I prescribe regular physical activity. Regular exercise combats fatigue within a week or two. Nearly everyone who begins regular physical activity appreciates the benefit of increased energy. Even daily tasks like doing the laundry or carrying groceries upstairs seem easier.

Exercising, then, is very much a "casting off of restraints." The sedentary life cannot be a healthy life. Moderate activity can yield enormous benefits, both in quantity and quality of life. Not only will it help you survive, it is absolutely necessary to thrive.

CHAPTER 8
CHANGING THE WAY WE EAT

Perhaps the most difficult behaviors to change are what we eat and the way in which we eat. Food is essential to the maintenance of life, necessary for the functioning of the human organism. Eating is behavior that creates rhythm to the cadence of our lives. Eating lies at the core of our cultural identity and as such is behavior deeply rooted in the social, psychological soil in which we attempt to survive and thrive. This behavior, however fundamental, is still just that: behavior. It is the outward expression of the dynamic interplay between our thoughts, bodies, and emotions. In fact, if the schema of the self that we discussed holds true, then it is precisely *because* food intake is so fundamental to biologic processes that this behavior is so profoundly and dynamically linked to our thoughts and emotions.

We see the extreme link between eating behavior and emotions and thoughts in eating disorders, such as anorexia nervosa and bulimia. Anorexia nervosa, a potentially fatal disorder, is the willful restriction of food intake (behavior) because of the fear of being overweight (emotion) and the belief that one's appearance is overweight (thought) even if the person is quite thin or even emaciated. Bulimia nervosa, a more common disorder than anorexia nervosa, involves the behavior of regular episodes of binge eating, followed by attempts to counteract the potential weight gain from that eating, usually by some form of purging through the use of laxatives or self-induced vomiting. The binge behavior is often associated with the sense of being out of control, followed by feelings of intense guilt or shame, often accompanied by feelings of depression and anxiety. Those with this disorder usually have obsessive thoughts of dissatisfaction with their bodies' shape or weight.

But these are the extremes. Those with these disorders are obviously in need of psychotherapy and other treatments. Much more common, however, is eating behavior that results in overweight and obesity, and eating behavior that fails to achieve the amount and kinds of nutrients that we now know can protect against disease. Over one-half of the adults in this country are overweight, meaning most people are eating far more calories than they need. We will explore the many reasons why this is so, but it must be said from the outset that this behavior clearly represents an expression of the interplay between our thoughts, our bodies, and our emotions. The pattern of this dynamic interplay is now embedded in our culture and modern society.

Though we usually think of the word "diet" to refer to some intentionally restrictive and regimented meal plan with the design of losing weight, it is important to realize that we all are "on" a diet. Our diets are simply what, when, and how much we usually eat. A diet is behavior. Eating well as a healthy behavior does involve intentions—and some restrictions—but a healthy diet should not be seen as a time-limited program of painful sacrifices which will one day "end" when a certain goal is reached. The word "diet" comes from the Greek *diaita*, which translates as "way of life." This root meaning of the word highlights just how fundamental eating behavior is to our lives. Through our diets—what, when, and how much we eat—we see the outward expression of the interplay between our bodies, minds, and emotions. To change this behavior, most of us will ultimately need to critically reflect on our thoughts and emotions. A healthy diet, then, is a healthy way of living.

It is important to note the emphasis on what is considered healthy or unhealthy. The food itself is not healthy or unhealthy. The behavior—in this case, the eating behavior—is what can be considered healthy or unhealthy. Though in this chapter we will go in to some detail about the content and the nutritional value of various foods, our focus should not be on the types of food, but on our behaviors. This focus will lead, ultimately, to the frequency and amount of food we eat. A healthy diet is a healthy way of living.

Eating well—and we will provide a framework for what that entails—leads to substantial health benefits. If we include loss of excess body weight in the results of eating well, a healthy diet can lead to substantial reductions in the risk of coronary heart disease, hypertension, stroke, diabetes, hypercholesterolemia, obesity, colon cancer, and gastric cancer. Again, we see in this short list the conditions responsible for the majority of the disease burden in our country. Later in this chapter, we will discuss specific kinds of foods that appear to be associated with reductions in risk of particular diseases, such as heart disease and colon cancer.

Throughout this chapter, though we will be focusing on eating well for health, it is important to keep in mind that eating is a source of genuine pleasure. Eating well involves behavior that is healthy and pleasurable. Can this be achieved? I believe it can, especially if we approach diet—our way of living—from the standpoint of how much and how often we eat certain foods, rather than focusing on the food itself. Yes, you can eat well and enjoy the chocolate cake!

Living Longer Working Stronger

Let's first consider eating well from the standpoint of the most basic physiologic function of food intake: providing energy for the proper function of our bodies. Energy can be quantified. The unit of measure we use to quantify the potential energy in food is the calorie. The term "calorie" comes from the Latin *calor*, which means "heat." One calorie is the amount of heat required to raise the temperature of one gram of water by one degree Celsius. When we use the term to refer to the amount of potential energy in food, we use the term Calorie, with a capital "C," which is actually a kilocalorie, or one-thousand calories, or the amount of energy required to raise one thousand grams (one kilogram) of water by one degree Celsius. When we apply the idea of the kilocalorie to humans in the context of weight management, it is useful to consider that, roughly speaking, one "pound" of a person has about 3500 kilocalories of potential energy. If we use up that 3500 kilocalories and do no replace it, we will lose that pound. If we take in 3500 kilocalories more than we use, we will gain one pound.

Food, then, is potential energy, which is released upon ingestion. That energy is used as needed to fuel the proper function and maintenance of the body's organ systems. If it is not needed, then the energy is stored. And that is where we can get into trouble.

The amount of energy we need—or the number of Calories we need to take in—is determined by two main factors. The primary factor is the energy required to maintain the body's resting functions, or *resting metabolism*. The other factor is physical activity, which makes our organ systems work harder, therefore requiring more energy. Resting metabolism is itself determined by genetic, environmental, and hormonal factors, and by *body mass*. This last contributor to resting metabolism, body mass, may be the most important as we consider how to eat well.

An imbalance between caloric intake and energy expenditure leads to overweight and obesity, or an unhealthy increase in body mass. That body mass, even (or especially) the excess body mass, is itself metabolically active, meaning it too requires energy to function. Those who are overweight and obese, and whose weight has been stable over time, are eating enough calories to maintain their weight. In this sense, they are not overeating, but are taking in the number of calories to maintain their weight, including their excess weight. But they have clearly taken in enough calories to increase their body mass over time and now maintain it. This is just one of the many vicious circles involved in being overweight: the body—the overweight or obese body—*needs* the number of calories taken in to maintain its function.

Nevertheless, if you are overweight or obese, you *are* overeating from a healthy living perspective. You are literally feeding your excess weight, and you are overfeeding your body's basic metabolic functions. So what is your "ideal body weight?"

There is no exact weight that is ideal for any given business professional. We can at best only provide a range of weights that are recommended or considered "ideal." These ranges are determined through epidemiologic studies of large populations of patients whose weights were compared to the presence or absence of health problems and mortality rates over time. Researchers identified the weight values that were associated with an increased risk of weight-related health problems, like high blood pressure, diabetes, and heart disease. Ideal body weight ranges are directly related to height, and are different for men and women. A rough estimate of your ideal body weight (in pounds) can be determined through a simple calculation:

For men: **50 + 2.3 (Height in inches – 60)**
For women: **45.5 + 2.3 (Height in inches –60)**

A more refined measure of the ideal body weight range takes into account estimates of excess body mass that is likely due to total body fat. This measure is called the Body Mass Index or BMI. Like the equations above, the BMI takes into account height. To determine your BMI, you can use the following equations:

Weight (lbs) x 703/ (height in inches)^2
        Or
Weight (kg)/ (height in meters)^2

Body Mass Index Table

To use the table, find the appropriate height in the left-hand column labeled Height. Move across to a given weight. The number at the top of the column is the BMI at that height and weight. Pounds have been rounded off.

BMI	19	20	21	22	23	24	25	26	27	28	29	30	31	32	33	34	35
Height (inches)	Body Weight (pounds)																
58	91	96	100	105	110	115	119	124	129	134	138	143	148	153	158	162	167
59	94	99	104	109	114	119	124	128	133	138	143	148	153	158	163	168	173
60	97	102	107	112	118	123	128	133	138	143	148	153	158	163	168	174	179
61	100	106	111	116	122	127	132	137	143	148	153	158	164	169	174	180	185
62	104	109	115	120	126	131	136	142	147	153	158	164	169	175	180	186	191
63	107	113	118	124	130	135	141	146	152	158	163	169	175	180	186	191	197
64	110	116	122	128	134	140	145	151	157	163	169	174	180	186	192	197	204
65	114	120	126	132	138	144	150	156	162	168	174	180	186	192	198	204	210
66	118	124	130	136	142	148	155	161	167	173	179	186	192	198	204	210	216
67	121	127	134	140	146	153	159	166	172	178	185	191	198	204	211	217	223
68	125	131	138	144	151	158	164	171	177	184	190	197	203	210	216	223	230
69	128	135	142	149	155	162	169	176	182	189	196	203	209	216	223	230	236
70	132	139	146	153	160	167	174	181	188	195	202	209	216	222	229	236	243
71	136	143	150	157	165	172	179	186	193	200	208	215	222	229	236	243	250
72	140	147	154	162	169	177	184	191	199	206	213	221	228	235	242	250	258
73	144	151	159	166	174	182	189	197	204	212	219	227	235	242	250	257	265
74	148	155	163	171	179	186	194	202	210	218	225	233	241	249	256	264	272
75	152	160	168	176	184	192	200	208	216	224	232	240	248	256	264	272	279
76	156	164	172	180	189	197	205	213	221	230	238	246	254	263	271	279	287

Source: NHBLI, http://www.nhlbi.nih.gov/guidelines/obesity/bmi_tbl.htm

A BMI of 18.5-24.9 kg/m^2 is considered normal weight. A BMI of 25-29.9 is considered overweight. And a BMI of greater than or equal to 30 is obese. It is important to note that the BMI overestimates total body fat in those who are very muscular, such as body builders. Those who are "obese" are at least 20-30 lbs overweight. It is at this degree of excess weight that the risk of health problems dramatically increases. In 2001, over one in five adult Americans was obese. And the numbers are rising by the year, in truly epidemic proportions. It is important to take the time to accurately assess your BMI. A survey of American adults, conducted in 1994, showed that among those who thought that their weight was "about right," 45% of men and nearly 20% of women had BMI values greater than or equal to 25. (1994 CSFII, USDA) This data indicates that many are at risk for weight related health problems and don't know it.

If your BMI is 25 or above, you are overweight. If you are continuing to gain weight, you are taking in more calories than you are using. Notice that we have not yet talked about *what* foods you are eating. For now, just realize that if you are overweight and gaining weight *you are taking in too many calories.*

Now, if you are overweight or obese and have been at the same weight for years at a time, you are taking in about as many calories as you are using. But you are feeding your own fat! You are taking in calories for your total body fat to utilize, not for your body's functions.

So how many calories do you need? About 60-70% of your daily caloric needs are determined by your resting metabolism, what scientists call the basal metabolic rate, or BMR. This value represents the number of calories to keep your body functioning at rest. This energy fuels normal function of the heart, lungs, kidneys, brain, and other body tissues. The BMR is dependent on weight, height, age, sex, and genetics. We can estimate the energy required to fuel your BMR through the use of yet another equation, the Harris Benedict equation, which was developed nearly a century ago. It is different for men and women:

Men: 66 + (13.7 X wt in kg) + (5 X ht in cm) - (6.8 X age in years) = kcal for BMR

Women: 655 + (9.6 X wt in kg) + (1.8 X ht in cm) - (4.7 X age in years) = kcal for BMR

Note: 1 inch = 2.54 cm.

1 kilogram = 2.2 lbs.

Consider the following example:

A 50 year old male, 5'10", who weighs 200 lbs.

$66 + (13.7 \times 91 \text{ kg}) + (5 \times 178 \text{ cm}) - (6.8 \times 50) = 1862 \text{ kcal}$

An easier equation for estimating the energy required to fuel the BMR was developed by the World Health Organization, and takes into account age, sex, and total body weight.

AGE	MALE	FEMALE
18-29	$(15.5 \times \text{lbs}/2.2) + 679$	$(14.7 \times \text{lbs}/2.2) + 496$
30-60	$(11.6 \times \text{lbs}/2.2) + 879$	$(8.7 \times \text{lbs}/2.2) + 829$
>60	$(13.5 \times \text{lbs}/2.2) + 487$	$(10.5 \times \text{lbs}/2.2) + 596$

To maintain his normal, resting bodily functions, this person requires 1862 kcal per day. If we use the WHO equation, the value is 1934 kcal, an amount within 100 kcal of the more complicated equation. But most sedentary people engage in at least some activity: bathing, eating, getting up and down from the sitting position, etc. This activity, however minimal, requires energy in the form of calories as well. We can account for energy needed for physical activity through the use of a multiplier value as follows:

Activity Multiplier

Sedentary = BMR X 1.2   (little or no exercise, desk job)
Lightly active = BMR X 1.375 (light exercise/sports 1-3 days/wk)
Mod. active = BMR X 1.55   (moderate exercise/sports 3-5 days/wk)
Very active = BMR X 1.725 (hard exercise/sports 6-7 days/wk)
Extr. active = BMR X 1.9   (hard daily exercise/sports & physical job or 2X day training, i.e., marathon, contest etc.)

To return to our example, if the 50-year-old male described above is sedentary, we multiply the value of the BMR by 1.2 to get 2234 kcal. That value is an *estimate* of the number of calories this person needs to maintain weight. As we will see when we consider the number of calories typically consumed in this country, it is very likely that our example patient is eating much more than 2200 kcal per day, and that he is continuing to gain weight.

The Harris-Benedict equation assumes a normal amount of total body fat and lean body mass. It must be stressed that body fat uses calories inefficiently compared to muscle. Therefore, the more muscle a body has, the higher its BMR. The more fat a person has, the lower the BMR, relative to someone with less body fat, but with the same body weight. The more obese a person is, the less accurate is the BMR calculation in terms of predicting what daily caloric needs are for a given business professional.

A less precise way to quickly calculate caloric requirements for adults, which takes into account both age, sex, and activity level, is as follows:

Obese or very inactive people	11 kcal/lb
Over 55, active women, sedentary men	13 kcal/lb
Active men or very active women	15 kcal/lb
Thin or very active men	20 kcal/lb

Calories Needed Daily Per Pound Based On Activity and Sex.

Activity Level	Women	Men
Very light	12	14
Light	13	15
Moderate	14	16
Strenuous	15	17
Very strenuous	16	18

As a guide to activity level, very light activity is sitting most of the day with up to two hours of standing or walking. A moderate activity includes housework, gardening, or carpentry. Examples of very strenuous activity are tennis, swimming, running, basketball, or football.

The values one gets from these quick calculations will approximate the values obtained through the use of the Harris-Benedict equation and the activity multiplier. I encourage you to make use of one of these equations to get a rough estimate of what your daily energy requirements are for maintaining weight, so that you might determine how many calories a day you should be eating. We will return to the issue of calories later in this discussion.

Eating well *begins* with taking in as many calories as one needs: achieving a balance between energy in—in the form of calories—and energy out— comprised of basal metabolic rate and physical activity. The staggering rate of rise in the prevalence of obesity clearly indicates that, as a country, we are eating much more than we need. That so many are actively gaining weight— even those who are already overweight—indicates that not only are they feeding their fat to maintain weight, they are also overfeeding their fat— taking in far more calories than necessary.

Data collected by the NHANES, bears this out. The average number of kilocalories per day consumed by American adults has risen from about 2000 in 1969 to 2700 in 1994. And the numbers continue to rise! Increasing one's caloric intake by 700 kcal per day, assuming physical activity remains the same, would result in a weight gain of about 1.5 lbs per week: almost 80 lbs a year!

That dramatic increase in energy intake would not be problematic if Americans were more physically active, but the data suggest that the opposite is true: We are more sedentary than ever. This reduction in physical activity decreases energy out—further tipping the scales (literally and figuratively) towards taking in too much.

What is responsible for this increase in energy intake? There are several forces at work, but a description of a patient of mine will capture at least three important factors. My patient is a business professional in his mid-30s and has been about 30 pounds overweight for the last 10 years. He is married with two children, and leads a typical, often frantic, suburban lifestyle. He gets no regular exercise, but is "active" to the point of feeling quite tired by the end of the day, due to the strains of a busy office practice and the activity associated with the children. He tells me that the refrigerator and cupboards in his kitchen are filled with "low fat," "lite," "healthy," and "diet" foods. He and his wife routinely buy these products instead of "regular" bread, ice cream, cheese, and other foods, with the expectation that they are "healthier" choices. Despite these dietary efforts, he continues to gain weight. In addition, because of perceived time constraints and the effort required to eat at home, they either eat out or eat take-out several times a week, especially for lunches.

My patient's situation is not at all unique or rare. The bottom line is that if he is gaining weight: He is eating more calories than he is using over time. A calorie is a calorie. It is a finite amount of energy consumed. The first factor at work in my friend's weight gain is the kind of food that is in his cupboards. The marketing strategies of the companies that make "low fat" and "lite" food products are nothing short of brilliant—and have proven widely successful. Though these products may indeed have a lower fat content, they do not differ much in the number of calories in any given portion. The American public has been buying and eating these products believing that the products themselves are "healthy," but they have in the process been eating more calories, under the illusion that "lite" means fewer calories. Most of these products, while low in fat, are supplemented with added sugars, which are simply carbohydrates that contain calories with little nutritional value. In fact, recent food intake surveys indicate that the *percent* of fat in the total diet of Americans has dropped over the last 20 years, but the *absolute amount* of fat has increased. We are eating more calories, so we continue to gain weight.

The second factor is portion size. We live in the "super-size" age, where portions of food eaten are getting larger and larger. This phenomenon was recently documented in a study published in the Journal of the American Medical Association. (Nielsen, Popkin, JAMA 2003; 289; 450-53). The researchers found that nearly all food portion sizes increased from 1977-78 to 1994-96, the period of time in which data was collected. Notably, salty snack portions increased by 60%, soft drinks by over 50%, and cheeseburgers by almost 30%. This trend is also seen with foods considered to be more "healthy," such as bagels and muffins. The size of these foods continues to grow. One large bagel has about the same number of calories as four slices of bread. Yet the perception is that it is "healthier" to eat the bagel. We will further discuss nutrient content below, but the basic fact of the increase in total number of calories must be taken seriously. It is, I believe, the primary reason for the weight gain seen in this country: not what one eats, but how much.

Not surprisingly, the same JAMA study found that the increase in portion size of foods was most dramatic in fast-food restaurants. The data collected in this study indicates that the total number of calories in a fast-food meal consisting of a soft drink, a cheeseburger, and French fries was about 1000 in the mid-1990s, up from 700 kcal in the mid-1970s. Experience in fast-food chains indicates that the number of calories in such a meal today is likely to be even higher.

The fact that portion sizes have increased in fast-food restaurants points to a third factor at work: Americans are eating out more than ever. A USDA survey of eating patterns in 1995 found that about 34% of American adults' total food intake came from "food away from home." That is up from 19% 20 years ago. Prepared foods are frequently higher in calories because of the way they are prepared in addition to the portion sizes. We are less likely to limit or restrict our food choices, either in the kind or amounts of food, when we go out to eat, and it is probable that we are more likely to drink alcohol and get dessert, all of which adds to an increase in the total number of calories.

At the beginning of this chapter we acknowledged the link between eating behavior and the interplay between the body, thoughts, and emotions. Overeating is linked to what I call "automatic" eating. This kind of eating is eating as a reflex: a non-deliberate behavior triggered by either an intense emotional state or other cues. The emotional states are usually low to moderate level anxiety states, often occurring when we are alone, and in the evening when the stressors of the day have "caught up to us." They frequently occur at work, during a break of some kind, when that kind of food is made available, either through a vending machine or local restaurant. Other cues are often social settings, like receptions or cocktail parties, which themselves can be associated with a variety of sources of anxiety, or other behaviors, such as watching television or a sporting event. This automatic, reflexive, non-deliberate kind of eating usually involves food that is high in calories and low in nutritional content. The bite-sized portions of food involved in this kind of eating do not allow for a real assessment of quantity (e.g., "How many handfuls of salted nuts did I eat?") Many people engage in this kind of eating at least once a day yet do not include it in their recollection of how much they typically eat.

Above all, eating well means eating as much as you need, depending on your basal metabolic rate and level of physical activity. It means not eating too much. Since being overweight and obese are the results of not eating well and confer the greatest risk, the most important goal is not to overeat.

Now that we have determined how much we need to eat well, it is time to turn to the much more complicated question of what we should eat. I want to stress that these two questions—how much and what kind of foods—are absolutely related. I don't want the discussion of the kinds of food to overshadow the more basic question of how much food it takes to eat well. It is my personal belief that most of the morbidity and mortality associated with dietary factors in this country is related to overeating, not what kind of foods we are eating. Many of the dietary fads seen today, which stress the importance of one kind of food group over another, are distractions from the more basic question of how much we are eating. As we shall see, there are elements of a diet which have important implications for specific health concerns, particularly relative to coronary heart disease. But too much of any food group can lead to over-feeding—feeding our fat instead of providing energy for the optimal function of our vital organs.

A balance must be struck between energy in and energy out, just like the accounting on a balance sheet. If you are overweight, you are eating too many calories compared to the number of calories that you burn each day.

It is the opinion of the American Dietetic Association and the U.S. Department of Agriculture that a "total diet approach" be utilized when discussing recommendations for healthy eating. I concur completely with this approach. A total diet approach means that certain kinds of food are not "good" or "bad" in themselves, but that the choices surrounding portion size and frequency of eating a particular food are what constitute healthy eating. The total diet approach is visually portrayed in the Food Guide Pyramid (see figure) provided by the U.S. Department of Agriculture.

The recommendations provided by the Food Guide Pyramid imply that one can approach healthy eating and include all kinds of food in one's diet. Recent success of diets which stress one food group over another ("eat no carbohydrates" vs. "eat no fat" vs. "never eat sugar") are not only unrealistic in terms of long-term adherence, but can result in eating habits that are unhealthy when one avoids certain food groups that actually provide important nutrients. In addition, many of these diets deny one of the most important aspects of eating: enjoyment. A piece of apple pie is simply delicious! Apple pie is not "bad" for you. It should not be considered a "guilty pleasure" or a "reward" for good behavior.

Let's consider the Food Guide Pyramid for a moment. The pyramid shape, of course, suggests that the foods at the bottom should make up more calories than the foods at the top. This distribution also implies that the bottom foods should be eaten with more frequency.

Living Longer Working Stronger

The Pyramid divides types of food into the following categories:

Bread, Cereal, Rice, and Pasta
Fruits
Vegetables
Milk, Yogurt, and Cheese
Meat, Beans, Eggs, and Nuts
Fats, Oils, and Sweets

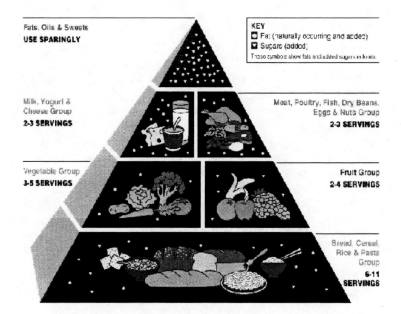

Source: USDA

The Pyramid provides not only a graphic representation of how much of each food group to eat, but also offers recommendations regarding actual quantities by listing the number of "servings" per day for each group. A range is provided, with the lower number roughly corresponding to a 1600 kcal/day diet and the higher number to a 2800 kcal/day diet.

Not surprisingly, Americans are not following this advice, especially with certain food groups. Table X1 provides some of the results of the last Continuing Survey of Food Intake by Individuals conducted by the USDA, which tracks eating patterns of our population periodically.

TABLE X1

	Recommended # of Servings	Actual # Male	Actual # Female
Grains	6-11	7.9	5.5
Vegetables	3-5	4.1	3.1
Fruit	2-4	1.5	1.5
Dairy	2-3	1.5	1.5
Meat, Beans, Eggs, and Nuts	5-7	6.4	3.9
Fats, Oils, Sweets	"sparingly"	39% of total calories	39% of total calories

Source: USDA CSFII, 1994-1996

A few issues regarding these results are worth mentioning. First, on average, adult women are consistently below recommended amounts of the various food groups, except for the fats, oils, and sweets category. We eat too few vegetable and fruits. Less than 25% of Americans even ate the minimum recommended amounts of fruits and vegetables, even for a 1600 kcal diet! (See table fruits). As we will discuss later, this fact alone has important health implications. The most glaring conclusion, however, is that nearly 40% of our caloric intake comes from the "tip" of the pyramid! We have turned the food pyramid on its head! What we are supposed to be eating very rarely— "sparingly," to quote the USDA—are foods making up well over a third of our energy on a daily basis. This is certainly one reason why America is getting fatter.

Percentage of Adults Who Reported Eating Fewer Than Five Servings of Fruits and Vegetables a Day, by Sex, 2000

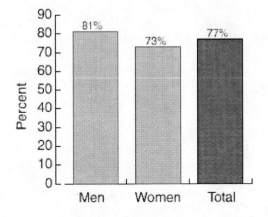

Source: CDC, Behavioral Risk Factor Surveillance System.

To get a better understanding of why we are not paying attention to these dietary recommendations and may, in fact, be doing just the opposite of what is recommended for healthy eating, we will need to review some nutritional concepts that will prove quite useful as we chart out a plan for eating well. The discussion that follows is somewhat detailed and includes some of the basic language of nutrition and biochemistry that is fundamental to an informed understanding of food and how we might better choose to eat well.

The food groups provided in the Pyramid are an attempt to name and group foods that we recognize into categories that roughly correspond to a more scientific grouping of types of food, which many readers will readily appreciate. The groups have familiar names and are called *carbohydrates*, *fats*, and *protein*. They all are absolutely essential to the proper growth and functioning of the human body. Consider the following food groups from the Pyramid and their corresponding energy source:

Carbohydrates

Carbohydrates are foods made up of carbon ("carbo-") and hydrogen ("hydrate") atoms and exist as either single molecules, pairs, or as longer chains of molecules, strung together by chemical bonds. *Simple carbohydrates*, or sugars, exist primarily as single or paired molecules and require little digestion to be absorbed from the intestine into the bloodstream. In our diets, the most abundant simple carbohydrates are fructose, found in fruit; lactose, found in milk; and sucrose, or table sugar, made from sugar cane. The most important simple carbohydrate is glucose, which exists as a single molecule, and is the molecule referred to by the term "blood sugar." Though not found alone in many foods, it is one of the basic building blocks for the more complex carbohydrates. Carbohydrates provide 4 kcal per gram.

The *complex carbohydrates* are primarily found in plants, including grains, fruits, and vegetables. There are two kinds: starch and cellulose. Both are made up of chains of glucose molecules, but these chains are arranged in such a way that starch can be broken down to glucose and absorbed into the blood stream, providing calories or energy for the body, but cellulose cannot. Cellulose is what makes up most of what we call *fiber* in the diet. Though it is a carbohydrate, fiber does not provide calories for energy, because it does not get absorbed from the intestine. As we shall see later, however, its presence in our diets serves very useful functions.

Protein

Protein is a food type made up of nitrogen-containing amino acids. The predominant food sources of protein in the American diet are meat, beans, and eggs. The variety of complex proteins we eat are digested or broken down in our intestines, then absorbed into the blood stream, where they are reassembled into the proteins necessary for the building and maintenance of nearly all of the body's organs and tissues, including muscles, brain, blood cells, and skin. Proteins make up hormones, antibodies, and enzymes, as well as the DNA molecules that carry the genetic code. The body can make most of the 22 amino acids from the breakdown products of ingested proteins and other foods. However, there are nine amino acids that the body cannot make on its own, and these amino acids, called the *essential amino acids*, must come from dietary protein. One gram of protein also contains 4 kcal of energy, the same amount as carbohydrates.

Fat

Dietary fats, like carbohydrates, are also made up of carbon and hydrogen atoms, but are arranged in such a way that they require special digestion to be absorbed from the intestine into the bloodstream. As a molecule, fats are energy-dense, carrying more than twice as much energy as carbohydrates or protein (9 kcal per gram). There are several kinds of dietary fats. All are found in most fat-containing foods. It is important to discern the *relative amounts* of these different kinds of fats in various foods. *Saturated fats* are fats that are saturated with hydrogen atoms. These fats consist primarily as solids at room temperature and are found in high amounts in butter, most cheeses, lard, bacon, and the "fat" in cuts of meat. Palm and coconut oils are saturated fats that are liquid at room temperature. The *unsaturated* fats, which have room for one (*monounsaturated*) or more (*polyunsaturated*) hydrogen atoms, exist predominantly as liquids at room temperature. Unsaturated fats are found in vegetable oils, such as corn, sunflower, and olive oil, as well as fish and plant food sources, such as soybeans and peanuts.

Like the amino acids, the body can manufacture most of the fat necessary for bodily functions, which, apart from energy storage, includes formation of cell membranes for all organs, including muscle and brain. But there are certain types of fat that must come from the diet. These are called the *essential fatty acids*, of which there are two: Linoleic acid, which is, because of its molecular configuration called an omega-6 fatty acid; and alpha-linolenic acid, an omega-3 fatty acid. Linoleic acid and the other omega-6 fatty acids are present in most vegetable oils; since these oils are used frequently in food preparation and in margarine, we usually get plenty of them in our diets. The alpha-linolenic acid and the other omega-3 fatty acids, however, are present in relatively small amounts in the typical American diet. Omega-3s are found in "fatty" fish, such as tuna, salmon, and trout, as well as certain plant oils, especially canola oil, walnut oil, and flaxseed oil. Olive oil is a rich source of monounsaturated oil, but not essential fatty acids. Knowing about these different kinds of fats is essential in making deliberate, sustained choices in our efforts to eat well.

Another kind of dietary fat, and for many Americans, a very common source of fat, is the *trans-fatty acids*. This kind of fat is the result of a chemical process which adds hydrogen (a process called *hydrogenation*) to liquid unsaturated fat, especially vegetable oils, making it turn into a solid or semi-solid. Fat in this form preserves the shelf-life of packaged food. Trans-fatty acids are present in large amount in store-bought baked goods, fried foods, stick margarine, and many other products. You can determine if these kinds of fat are present in a food by looking at the ingredients label. If you see "partially hydrogenated vegetable oil," any type of oil that is "hydrogenated," or "vegetable shortening," the food contains trans-fatty acids. They are hard to avoid in an American diet.

There is much more to say regarding dietary fat and making proper food choices. We will return to the topic as we chart our plan for eating well.

Let's get back to the Food Guide Pyramid, with what we now know about the kinds of food that are available to us. We can see that the predominant source of carbohydrates, including fiber, comes from the Grain, Fruit, and Vegetable groups. Most of the protein that Americans get comes from the Meat, Bean, and Egg group. And most of the fat comes from—the fat group. Though we are to ingest fats and oils (liquid fats) "sparingly," these energy sources, along with added sugars, make up nearly 40% of the average American diet. How are we getting all of this dietary fat and added sugar? A careful look at the Nutrition Facts Label, which is now present on nearly all packaged foods, will help answer that question.

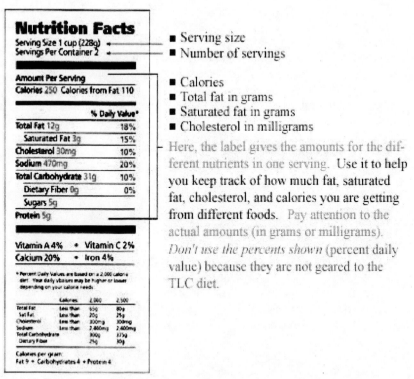

Source: http://www.nhlbi.nih.gov/chd/Tipsheets/readthelabel.htm

The Nutrition Facts Label, a joint effort by the U.S. Department of Agriculture and the Food and Drug Administration, standardized and mandated in 1994, must now be visible on nearly all packaged, store-bought food. As we shall see, the information on that label is linked directly to the recommendations in the Food Guide Pyramid. Though the food nutrition label contains valuable information that can help an informed purchaser make healthy food choices, there are elements of the food label, which can be quite misleading.

Consider the example of the food label seen on the previous page. See the first line, which provides the "serving size" used to calculate the nutritional contents of the product. "Serving size" is a concept taken from the Food Guide Pyramid, which, if you go back to the FGP diagram, provides how much of each food group is recommended on a daily basis, by means of the number of "servings" per day. The important point here, however, is that considering food in terms of "servings" is *not* actually how we eat. Why? Because a "serving" is not a "helping" or a "portion": terms we use to describe what we actually consume in a typical American meal. In fact, a "serving" is usually quite less than what most people consider a "helping" to be. An example will help clarify this very important nutritional concept.

Consider a typical spaghetti dinner, including a plate of pasta, some garlic bread, the sauce, and a few meatballs. If we look at the Food Guide Pyramid, we might think our dinner has added up to the following servings from the various food groups:

One serving from the Grains group for the spaghetti.
One serving from the Grains group for the bread.
One serving from the Vegetable group for the sauce.
One serving from the Meat group for the meatballs.

There you have it: a well-balanced meal, with two Grains, one Vegetable, and one Meat. That leaves plenty of room for the lunch you had: a ham sandwich, a small bag of chips, and an iced tea, as well as the breakfast you had, which included a bagel with cream cheese, a glass of orange juice, and, well, yes, you did have that doughnut that somebody brought to work.

But a serving is *not* a helping. In fact, consider the following actual number of servings in that spaghetti dinner:

Spaghetti Dinner:

Food	Your portion	One Pyramid serving	Pyramid food group	Number of Pyramid servings you ate
Spaghetti	2 cups	½ cup	Grains	4
Garlic bread	2 slices	1 slice	Grains	2
Tomato sauce	1 cup	½ cup	Vegetables	2
Meatballs	6 oz.	2-3 oz.	Meat and beans	2-3

Source: USDA "How Much are You Eating?: Putting the Guidelines into Practice"; March 2002; Center for Nutrition Policy and Promotion; USDA; Home and Garden Bulletin 267-1

Refer back to the Food Guide Pyramid. You can see that this one spaghetti dinner brought you into the recommended number of servings *for a whole day* in both the Grains and Meat group. Any more meat that day and you would have exceeded the recommended number of daily servings!

So how much is a serving? The following table provides some examples.

WHAT COUNTS AS A SERVING?
Bread, Cereal, Rice, and Pasta Group (Grains Group)—whole grain and refined

- 1 slice of bread
- About 1 cup of ready-to-eat cereal
- 1/2 cup of cooked cereal, rice, or pasta

Vegetable Group

- 1 cup of raw leafy vegetables
- 1/2 cup of other vegetables cooked or raw
- 3/4 cup of vegetable juice

Fruit Group

- 1 medium apple, banana, orange, pear
- 1/2 cup of chopped, cooked, or canned fruit
- 3/4 cup of fruit juice

Milk, Yogurt, and Cheese Group (Milk Group)*

- 1 cup of milk** or yogurt**
- 1 1/2 ounces of natural cheese** (such as Cheddar)
- 2 ounces of processed cheese** (such as American)

Meat, Poultry, Fish, Dry Beans, Eggs, and Nuts Group (Meat and Beans Group)

- 2-3 ounces of cooked lean meat, poultry, or fish
- 1/2 cup of cooked dry beans[#] or 1/2 cup of tofu counts as 1 ounce of lean meat
- 2 1/2-ounce soyburger or 1 egg counts as 1 ounce of lean meat
- 2 tablespoons of peanut butter or 1/3 cup of nuts counts as 1 ounce of meat

Living Longer Working Stronger

For those who don't have an intuitive sense of the actual size of certain measured quantities, consider the following as further tips for appreciating serving size:

- 1 teaspoon (5 ml)
    - o about the size of the top half of your thumb
- 1 ounce (28 g)
    - o approximately inch cube of cheese
    - o volume of four stacked dice
    - o slice of cheese is about the size of a 3 1/2 inch computer disk
    - o chunk of cheese is about as thick as 2 dominoes
    - o 1 handful (palm) of nuts
- 2 ounces (57 g)
    - o 1 small chicken leg or thigh
    - o 1/2 cup of cottage cheese or tuna
- 3 ounces (85 g)
    - o serving of meat is about the size of a deck of playing cards
    - o 1/2 of whole chicken breast
    - o 1 medium pork chop
    - o 1 small hamburger
    - o unbreaded fish fillet
- 1/2 cup (118 ml)
    - o fruit or vegetables can fit in the palm of your hand
    - o about the volume of a tennis ball
- 1 cup (236 ml)
    - o about the size of a woman's fist
    - o breakfast cereal goes halfway up the side of a standard cereal bowl
    - o broccoli is about the size of a light bulb
- 1 medium apple = A tennis ball

(Adapted from www.exrx.net/Nutrition/FoodPortions.html)

The issue of serving size goes to the heart of the question of how Americans are gaining weight in the face of an information explosion regarding the nutritional value of food. We are eating more calories because we are eating larger portion sizes. The information on the Nutrition Facts label corresponds to serving size, but not portion or helping size. Again, consider a generously sized bagel. That is *four* servings from the Grain group (about four slices of bread).

Dr. Kevin Fosnocht

I suggest you go to your refrigerator or cupboard and take out a few items, such as a cereal box, a can of nuts, or some packaged cheese, and make your own assessment of how many "servings" per day you are currently eating. You may be surprised to discover that you are eating four servings of cereal at one sitting, or three servings of cheese with one sandwich (which would be the full recommended amount of dairy servings for the entire day). Along with these ample portions come many servings—and with many servings come the calories, which brings us to the next stop on the Nutrition Facts Label.

The food label provides the number of calories per serving, and this fact must always be kept in mind as one determines the caloric content of food. For example, a can of cashews may say that one serving is 200 calories. But one serving is typically one ounce: which is about 10 cashews. Two handfuls could be as many as 600 calories!

When patients come to me for dietary advice for weight loss, and I ask them to recount their meals for me over the last couple of days, invariably they underestimate how much they eat. They are not being deceitful. They are misinformed. In addition, we have grown accustomed to very large portion sizes and now, I believe, take them for granted. We expect to see portions bigger, and this is confirmed by the study mentioned earlier that has documented this trend: especially in restaurants. In fact, many people are eating about 30% more calories than they might think, and this misperception is usually due to a lack of understanding of portion size and the attendant calories. Many of my patients are eating well over 3000 kcal per day, even when they are not snacking or eating desserts, but report meals such as this:

Breakfast: cereal with banana, milk, coffee; eaten at home
Lunch: tuna sandwich, chips, iced tea; purchased at a local sandwich shop
Dinner: spaghetti with meatballs, garlic bread, two beers; eaten at home

If this person eats a large bowl of cereal with a large banana, whole milk, and adds sugar to his coffee, he has very likely consumed about 1100 kcal.

If the lunch consists of a tuna salad hoagie (on a medium roll), a "super-sized" bag of potato chips, and a large bottle of sweetened iced tea: 1500 kcal.

If this person is a 50-year-old, overweight (not obese) man who is sedentary, he has already exceeded the daily caloric requirements for weight maintenance (about 2400 kcal; see page L). In fact, the number of calories in this breakfast and lunch would be appropriate for a 35-year-old male of ideal body weight who runs 4 miles three times a week (about 2600 kcal).

If you add the spaghetti dinner, bread, and two beers: another 1800 kcal. The grand total: 4400 kcal! That's without snacking and without desserts. This patient continues to gain weight because he continues to exceed the number of calories he needs.

Let's reconsider the three meals above in the context of the recommended number of servings of each food group. Recall that the Food Guide Pyramid provides a range of recommended servings for each food group. The lower end of the range roughly corresponds to a diet of 1600 kcal per day, the higher end to a diet of about 2800 kcal per day.

This person is exceeding the recommended number of servings in both the Grain and Meat groups, even for the higher end calorie diet of 2800 kcal per day. His number of servings from the Fruits, Vegetables, and Dairy group are on the low end. He has a substantial amount of fat and added sugars, considering the amount of sugar in the iced tea, the mayonnaise and oil on the sub, and the butter and oil consumed at dinner. This latter Group is often "hidden" in the meals we eat—especially the prepared foods we purchase (notice that the greatest contribution to this food group came from the vendor-bought lunch).

And there you have the average American diet: high in grain-based carbohydrates and added sugars, protein from meat sources, and fats used to prepare foods; low in fruits, vegetables, and dairy products other than cheese. One does not need to count individual calories to see that this diet, however typical, is an example of not eating well on a few counts. For one, there are simply too many carbohydrates, including added sugars, and these carbohydrates have little fiber, the "other" kind of carbohydrate found in fruits and vegetables that does not add calories to the diet. For that reason, this diet does not represent the "total diet approach" necessary for eating well: there are too few of certain kinds of food. And lastly, eating well means being informed and aware of the "hidden" calories, especially the added fats and sugars used so often and in great quantities in prepared, packaged foods.

Let's return to the Nutrition Facts Label and let it guide our discussion.

We are going to discuss dietary fat content in some detail, as misconceptions regarding dietary fat (as well as dietary carbohydrates) are playing a role in the obesity and diabetes epidemics. (You may want to refer back to the "fats" section at the beginning of this chapter.)

As a society, we have labeled fat containing food as "bad" or "unhealthy" food, and "low fat" and "lite" foods as "good" or "healthy." This labeling is largely the result of marketing strategies, which have quite successfully billed these "low fat" foods as "healthy alternatives." Companies marketing such foods, however, have taken their cue, and in fact received popular legitimacy, from the Food Guide Pyramid's dietary recommendations which have grouped "fats, oils, and added sugars" into a single category that should be eaten "sparingly."

But thinking of foods in dualistic terms as "fat" and "carbs" will not allow for healthy eating. All fats are not the same, nor are all carbs, and their differences can have important health implications.

Look back to the Nutrition Facts Label. Next to the total calories value is the "calories from fat" value. This number tells you how many of the total calories are coming from fat. The current recommendation on the Nutrition Facts Label is that the number of calories per day you get from dietary fat should not exceed 30% of your total calories per day. A quick assessment of the label will tell you what percent of the calories in that food come from fat. But, as we've said already, total fat is not the whole story.

The next section of the Nutrition Facts Label provides a breakdown of the various nutrients in one serving of the food, again, beginning with fat. Now the label shows the amount of fat in grams. Recall that fat has 9 kcal per gram, so, in this case, the 12 grams of fat yield about 110 calories. Next to each nutrient is the "% DV," which means "percent daily value," a number that indicates what percent of the recommended amount of that type of nutrient is contained in a single serving of the food, *based on a 2000 kcal per day diet.* This last point is an important one. If you are a 130 lb, 25-year-old sedentary woman, your daily caloric needs are about 1700 kcal/day. So these amounts need to be interpreted in light of how many calories you actually need. To help keep track of the percentages and total values, the label has a "footnote" table which indicates the total recommended amount (in grams and milligrams) of the various nutrients for a 2000 kcal per day diet.

The current recommended daily intake of fat is less than 30% of total calories. The average American diet is about 37-40% of total calories. The major food sources of fat in the American diet are added fats, such as spreads, cooking oils, and salad dressings, as well as red meat and whole dairy products. Diets high in total fat have been shown in numerous studies to increase the risk of heart disease and cancer, particularly colon cancer and breast cancer. Limiting total fat intake can reduce your risk of developing these conditions.

The total fat value is then broken down, always to the amount of "saturated fat," and often to "monounsaturated" and "polyunsaturated." Here is where the real message regarding fat content in food lies, so if the nutritional information up to this point has been less than exciting for you, pay attention.

We now know that different types of fat appear to have different effects on one of the major determinants of heart disease risk: cholesterol. It must be appreciated from the start, that cholesterol is an essential molecule for the body, serving several important functions. It is the molecular precursor for hormones; it serves to make cell membranes function optimally; and it is used by the liver to make digestive substances called bile acids, stored and secreted by the gall bladder, which are necessary for the absorption of fat from the intestine into the blood stream. As is the case with most things, however, getting the right amount of cholesterol is a matter of degree. Too much cholesterol can lead to blocked arteries, especially in the heart. These blockages are what lead to heart attacks and strokes.

The cholesterol in our bodies comes either by eating cholesterol in foods or by being manufactured by the liver using—fats. Foods high in cholesterol are generally foods from animals, such as meat, shell fish, eggs (it's the yolk that has the cholesterol), and butter. The different types of dietary fat have been shown to have different effects on cholesterol, and it is strongly believed that these cholesterol effects can change the risk of developing heart disease. Let's review the different kinds of fat and how they change cholesterol.

The term cholesterol refers to a group of molecules called "lipoproteins." They are made up of a fat ("lipo-") molecule and a protein molecule. We divide the primary types of cholesterol into high-density lipoprotein (HDL) and low-density lipoprotein (LDL). HDL has come to be known as the "good" cholesterol: It protects against heart disease when elevated and increases the risk of developing heart disease when it is too low. LDL, or "bad" cholesterol, does just the opposite: When elevated it dramatically increases the risk of developing heart disease, and when low reduces that risk.

Through large epidemiologic studies, scientists have concluded a few effects that the various kinds of fat have on these two kinds of cholesterol. The ultimate effect, of course, is a change in the risk of developing heart disease. The Table below depicts the effects that the various kinds of fats have on HDL and LDL levels.

	HDL	LDL
Saturated fat	Increase	Increase
Monounsaturated fat	Increase	Decrease
Polyunsaturated fat	Increase	Decrease
Trans-fat	Decrease	Increase

As you can see, all types of fat except for the trans-fats can raise HDL levels. That's the good news. The bad news begins with saturated fat: It can dramatically increase LDL levels. It is for this reason that saturated fats are considered the real culprit in the American diet. Diets high in saturated fat have been consistently shown to be associated with higher rates of heart attacks than diets that have lower amounts of saturated fat. As a result, the Nutrition Facts Label clearly identifies the amount of saturated fat that is in each food. At present the nutrition recommendations on the label state that the number of calories per day that come from saturated fat should be no more than 10% of total calories. For a 2000 kcal diet, that's about 20g per day.

Many foods that you purchase will have a further breakdown of dietary fats, including the monounsaturated and polyunsaturated fats, on their Nutrition Facts Label. As you can see in the table, both of these types of fat can raise HDL levels and decrease LDL levels. That fact argues *for* fat in the diet. Recall that these fats are found in olive oil, canola oil, peanuts and fish such as salmon, tuna, and trout. Current nutritional thinking is that foods like these and their fats should be increased in the American diet. However, as we have noted before, these foods, because they are fats, are *energy dense*, meaning they have a lot of calories. Simply increasing the number of calories that come from unsaturated fats, without limiting total calories, will result in excess caloric intake and weight gain. Later we will discuss how to replace calories from carbohydrates, with calories from unsaturated fats.

Finally, let's consider trans-fats. Recall that these are fats found in most packaged baked goods, such as cookies and crackers, in stick margarine and in many fast foods and fried foods. Any food that has in its ingredients "partially hydrogenated" or "shortening" has trans-fats. Trans-fats are found especially in many "low-fat" foods. Though the label may indicate that the food is low in total fat, or even saturated fat, many of these foods have trans-fats.

These fats may have the worst effect on cholesterol values of all the different kinds of fat. They both decrease HDL and increase LDL: a double-whammy! Though I have repeatedly said that there are no "bad" foods, just bad choices, I can almost make an exception here. This kind of fat should simply be avoided. Now, it is nearly impossible in a modern diet to avoid tran-fats altogether. It is simply not realistic. But with deliberate, sustained choices, you can make informed decisions about how frequently you eat foods containing these fats.

At present, the Nutrition Facts Label does not directly tell us about trans-fats. There are plans for this to change, as government agencies recognize the health effects of these kinds of fat. For now, inspecting the ingredients list on the package will tell you if that food has this type of fat. If the label supplies you with the amount of saturated and unsaturated fat, like in our example, and the sum of those two values does not add up to the total fat count, then the difference represents the amount of trans-fat contained in a serving of the food.

It is safe to assume that most doughnuts and fried foods purchased in fast-food restaurants are cooked in fats containing high amounts of trans-fat. McDonald's, ever the supreme marketing strategist, announced in September 2002, that it plans to dramatically change the way its fried foods, especially French fries, are prepared. They now plan to use oils that have nearly half the amount of trans-fat and over twice the amount of polyunsaturated fat. Their fries will still be energy dense: the total amount of fat will remain the same, and therefore the total number of calories will remain the same, but in terms of content, this change *will* represent the opportunity to make a healthier choice in the fast-food arena.

Let's continue down the Nutrition Facts Label. Next on the list is the amount of *cholesterol* contained in a single serving of the food. As mentioned earlier, though the body manufactures most of the cholesterol it needs on a daily basis, we do get some directly from the diet. Here, the current recommendations are absolute amounts per day, as opposed to a percentage of total calories. The current recommendations for the general public are no more than 300mg per day. In our example, since one serving supplies 30mg of cholesterol, that comes to 10% of the daily value.

Why are eggs and cholesterol associated in our minds? Because one egg contains about 200mg of cholesterol! The cholesterol is found in the yolk of the egg. The egg white has no cholesterol.

The next item on the label is sodium. Sodium is a mineral that exists in food primarily as sodium chloride or "salt," so when we talk of salt content, we are talking about sodium content, and vice-versa. The recommended daily allowance of sodium is 2400mg per day. The typical American diet, however, includes between 3500 and 4000mg per day! The chief concern with so much salt in the food is its effect on blood pressure. Numerous studies have demonstrated that diets higher in salt are associated with higher blood pressures and that reducing dietary salt intake significantly lowers blood pressure, especially in patients who have mildly elevated blood pressure to begin with. Since high blood pressure, or hypertension, is one of the major risk factors for coronary artery disease, stroke, and kidney disease, maintaining a diet within the limits of the recommended amounts of sodium can help reduce the risk of these common, preventable diseases.

One problem is that about 70% of the salt that Americans get in their diets comes from the salt that is already in the food they have purchased, either packaged food or food bought in restaurants. That means we need to be make deliberate choices about what foods to eat if we are to control the amount of salt we take in.

Let's consider the next item on the Nutrition Facts Label—another very commonly heard but misunderstood word: carbohydrates. We have already discussed the different carbohydrates, the primary ones being sugars, (like sucrose, or table sugar, and fructose), starch, and fiber. The first two provide calories that the body uses for energy. The third, fiber, is not absorbed into the blood stream but serves other important functions in the diet. The recommendation from the USDA is that approximately 50-60% of calories should come from carbohydrates. Without even realizing it, many people are getting far more. This may be the result of "low fat" or "reduced fat" foods. The average businessman or woman may think he or she is eating "healthier" foods, usually with the hope of losing weight or not gaining weight, but in fact is eating the same number of calories. Consider a favorite snack of mine, fig cookies. Two "fat free" cookies contain 102 kcal. Two regular fig cookies contain 111 kcal—a trivial difference. Another example—again related to snack food where many Americans are getting a lot of calories—is frozen yogurt. A cup of "nonfat" frozen yogurt will contain 200 kcal, but a regular whole milk frozen yogurt will be 104 kcal. Why is this "low" and "non-fat" food not less in calories? You guessed it: It has more carbohydrates!

The Nutrition Facts Label must contain the amount for the total number of carbohydrates, as well as the amount of fiber and sugar. Why? Because the absolute amount of these two types of carbohydrates have important health implications. Let's consider sugar first.

In the last two decades, there has been an explosion in the consumption of added sugars. In 1997, the average American adult consumed about 33 teaspoons of sugar per day. That is nearly three times the recommended number of 10-12 teaspoons a day. One of the reasons is that so much of our food is now processed and packaged. In particular, "high fructose corn syrup" is now used as a sweetener in many products, including store-bought bread and cereals and is the chief sweetener in soft drinks and processed fruit juices. (The typical 12-ounce soft drink or fruit punch includes eight to 10 teaspoons of sugar!) If you go to your cupboard and begin examining the ingredients, you will be surprised to see how frequently this type of sugar is added to certain foods.

A 1998 study called "Coronary Artery Risk Development In Young Adults" demonstrated that the higher the sugar intake, the lower the HDL or good cholesterol concentrations. There are also several studies indicating that diets high in sugar are associated with elevations in triglyceride levels. Triglycerides are another component of cholesterol and high levels are associated with stroke and heart attack.

Choosing foods high in added sugars on a regular basis is not eating well because these foods typically have little to no nutritional value *other than providing calories*. The simple sugars found in fruit, milk, and vegetables carry with them important other nutrients, especially vitamins, minerals, and, very importantly—fiber. That leads us to our next step on the Nutrition Facts Label.

Recall that fiber (also referred to as "roughage" or "bulk") is a carbohydrate but it is not absorbed by the intestine and therefore does not provide energy. Fiber comes from plants, including fruits, vegetables, beans, and whole grains. (Note: the "whole" in "whole grains" is important: processed grains, such as white rice or the grains used to make white bread, have the fiber essentially removed, leaving only digestible carbohydrates in the form of starch). Americans typically consume about 10 to15 grams of fiber per day, which is much less than the recommended 25 to 30 grams per day. Why is so much recommended? A few reasons.

By not being digested, fiber stays in and moves through the intestine. Its presence in the intestine slows the absorption of sugars and fats into the blood stream; it binds bile acids (which are made of cholesterol) in the colon so that they are excreted, making the liver use its cholesterol stores to make more bile acid, which in turn lowers the circulating cholesterol levels. Fiber decreases the time it takes food to travel through the intestine, and it is this increased "transit time" that is thought to play a role in minimizing exposure of the colon to potentially toxic substances, thereby decreasing the risk of colon cancer.

There is mounting epidemiologic evidence linking high fiber diets and a reduced risk of developing colon cancer, and some other cancers. These studies looked at entire diets, not just the amount of fiber: Since diets high in fiber tend to be low in fat, it is not entirely clear what the active element in risk reduction is—high fiber content or low fat content. It may be both.

Finally, diets higher in fiber are also associated with a lower risk of development of coronary artery disease, largely due to the effect fiber has on cholesterol: It lowers total cholesterol and LDL, the so-called "bad cholesterol."

The next item on the Nutrition Facts Label is *protein*, another essential component to any diet. Foods rich in protein are meat, poultry, eggs, fish, and beans, but basically any food that was "living"—plant or animal---and is eaten "whole" will have protein in it. Protein carries 4 kcal/gram, the same as carbohydrates. If we eat more protein than our bodies require, this protein is metabolized to stored energy—fat. You will notice that the Nutrition Facts Label does not have a "%DV" value next to it. This is because it is assumed that protein will "make up" the rest of the caloric total, assuming fat comprises no more than 30% of daily calories and carbohydrates about 60%. That leaves protein at roughly 10% of the total. In the American diet, which has relatively large amounts of meat, getting enough protein in the diet is not difficult.

The last part of the Nutrition Facts Label provides an assessment of the percent of the recommended daily intake of two vitamins: Vitamin A and C; and two minerals: Iron (Fe) and calcium. We will discuss these nutrients later.

In 2000, the American Heart Association published dietary guidelines based on the latest scientific data about the effects of nutrition on coronary heart disease and its risk factors (like high blood pressure and high cholesterol). These guidelines centered on recommendations designed to prevent heart disease in people with both general and high risk for future cardiac events, such as heart attack and sudden death. The guidelines reflect a more refined understanding of the different types of fat and carbohydrates that we discussed above. In my opinion, though the recommendations are primarily meant for those at a higher risk for heart disease than the "average" person, they would benefit the average person as well. If we consider that over 60% of Americans are overweight, that 30% are obese, that 25% of adults in this country have high blood pressure, 25% are completely sedentary and 20% have the metabolic syndrome, then these recommendations will apply to a large number of people. In a primary care practice such as mine, where *nearly 70% of the women are obese (BMI > 30)*, then you can see how frequently I must dispense this advice. Let's consider some of the specific recommendations of the guidelines, then return to the Food Guide Pyramid to help chart out a plan for eating well.

TLC Diet in ATP III

Nutrient	Recommended Intake as Percent of Total Calories
Total Fat[1]	25-35%
Saturated	Less than 7%
Polyunsaturated	Up to 10%
Monounsaturated	Up to 20%
Carbohydrate[2]	50-60% of total calories
Protein	Approximately 15%
Cholesterol	Less than 200 mg per day
Total Calories[3]	Balance energy intake and expenditure to maintain desirable body weight and prevent weight gain

1. The 25-35% fat recommendation allows for increased intake of unsaturated fat in place of carbohydrates in people with the metabolic syndrome or diabetes.
2. Carbohydrate should come mainly from foods rich in complex carbohydrates. These include grains (especially whole grains), fruits and vegetables.
3. Daily energy expenditure should include at least moderate physical activity (contributing about 200 Kcal a day).
4. Options include adding 10-25 grams of viscous (soluble) fiber; 2 g/day of plant-derived sterols or stanols. Soy protein may be used as a replacement for some animal products.

Source: http://www.americanheart.org/presenter.jhtml?identifier=4764

Based on these guidelines, I recommend the following steps.

Step I: Determine your caloric needs based on desirable weight and energy expenditure.

Use the equations provided at the beginning of this chapter to determine your caloric needs. Most moderately active people will require approximately 1800 to 2800 kcal per day. This range is wide so it is important to determine what your needs are. If you exceed your caloric needs, you will gain weight. If you are overweight or obese now, you are exceeding your caloric needs for a desirable weight.

Step II: Determine an upper limit of *caloric* carbohydrate intake.

Make it between 50 and 60%. I recommend aiming for 50%. It should not exceed 60%. Diets high in carbohydrates can raise triglyceride levels, lower HDL levels, and put you at risk for not getting adequate amounts of the essential fatty acids found in food sources rich in unsaturated fat.
Carbohydrates should come primarily from whole foods and foods rich in complex carbohydrates, such as whole grains, fruits, and vegetables.

If you stick to this limit of carbohydrate intake and achieve your daily caloric goal, you will see that it is necessary is for you to *substitute* the number of calories you get from foods high in caloric carbohydrates with foods high in fiber, fat, and protein. This substitution process is the key to eating well and the expected results are improved cholesterol values and even a reduced risk of coronary heart disease.

Step III: Determine your upper limit of saturated fat intake, in grams, based on a value less than 7% of total calories.

I find it easier to think in fat based on grams, as opposed to an absolute number of calories. Use this equation to determine the number of grams of saturated fat that is your upper limit:

Total calories X .07/9 = # of grams saturated fat per day.

Step IV: Determine your goal of unsaturated fat intake, in grams, based on a value of 25% of total calories.

A similar equation can be used to determine this value:

Total calories X 0.25/9 = # of grams unsaturated fat per day.

The important point here is that *trans-fats* are considered unsaturated fat and at present do not appear on the Nutrition Facts Label. The average American eats about 5 grams of trans-fat a day and does not realize it, because it exists in processed and fried foods. Since current regulations require only total fat and saturated fat listings, do not assume that the food does not contain trans-fats. Again, you will have to go to the ingredients list and look for the trans-fat "code words": "partially hydrogenated," "hydrogenated," and "shortening."

In the American diet, unsaturated fats are primarily found in fish, nuts, and in oils such as olive and canola. Margarine has unsaturated fat, but stick margarine is high in trans-fats and should be avoided, given the many alternatives.

Step V: Try to get 25-30 grams a fiber per day.

Doing so will likely prove difficult for you if you eat a typical American diet already. Again, the principle of food substitution is important here. Food choices that include whole foods will increase fiber intake. White bread typically has no fiber, whereas whole wheat bread typically has 2g of fiber per slice. A cup of white rice may have 1g of fiber, but a cup of brown rice has about 4g. A cup of Kellogg's Corn Flakes has 0g of fiber, but a cup of Kellogg's All-bran Extra Fiber has 26g! How do they compare in calories? About equal.

Besides the direct health benefits of high fiber food choices, such as reduction in heart disease risk and cancer risk, these foods may help in keeping your total calories per day within your goal range. This is because fiber, though it increases the speed with which food travels through the intestine, *decreases* the time it takes for the stomach to empty the food just eaten. This makes you feel more "full" and you may be less likely to eat more calories.

Step VI: Determine the number of grams of protein per day, in grams, based on a value of 15% of total calories.

The following equation can be used:

Total calories X 15%/4 = # of grams of protein per day.

Most of the protein in the typical American diet comes from red meat sources, which are high in saturated fat. Poultry without the skin is much lower in saturated fat, provided the white meat is eaten. More than half the calories in typical hamburger meat come from fats, while white turkey meat has about 8% from fat. Their comparative protein content? About the same.

Besides meat, other high protein foods low in saturated fat are egg whites, beans, soy products, and fish.

Step VII: Limit dietary cholesterol to less than 200mg per day.

Eggs and butter are the chief sources of dietary cholesterol in our diets. This daily cholesterol limit means no more than seven eggs per week and argues for using non-stick, trans-fat free margarine in place of butter.

Step VIII: Limit daily sodium intake to 2400mg per day.

Since most of the salt we get comes not from what we add with the salt shaker but from purchased, processed, packaged food, we need to educate ourselves about salt content. For example, though soup is a food low in calories, a typical serving of Campbell's chicken noodle soup would provide nearly 1800mg of sodium. That amount of intake in a serving is not in itself problematic, but it means that consideration needs to be given to sodium intake throughout the rest of the day.

Consider these values your standards for daily consumption and make use of the Nutrition Facts Label to make food choices. But consider these values "average" values over the course of a given week. This will allow for flexibility in your food choices from day to day. Remember, foods are not healthy or unhealthy, but behavior can be either. For example, if you had 30 grams of saturated fat one day because of the hot dog, hamburger, and apple pie a la mode served at the family cook-out, over the next few days you should make food choices including far fewer amounts of saturated fat. This kind of averaging can be achieved with practice—you will get a feel for how much of certain types of food energy sources you have eaten. But realize that doing so requires deliberate choices. Eating well is behavior, and healthy behaviors absolutely require critical reflection.

We began this discussion of food choices based on the Food Guide Pyramid. We said that this kind of food guide represented a "total diet approach" to eating well. We then dissected the various types of food and are left with quite specific recommendations about the amounts of kinds of food that promote health. Let's return to the Food Guide Pyramid and see if the various recommendations "add up."

The Table below provides an estimation of the number of servings per day depending on the total caloric intake. *It is important to note that these estimates assume that food choices are involving lean cuts of meat and low fat dairy products.*

Table 1—Food Guide Pyramid Serving Recommendations

| Food group | Sample diets | | |
	1,600 calories	2,200 calories	2,800 calories
	Number of servings per day		
Grain group	6	9	11
Vegetable group	3	4	5
Fruit group	2	3	4
Dairy group[1]	2-3	2-3	2-3
Meat group (ounces)	5	6	7
Total fat (grams)[2]	53	73	93
Added sugars (teaspoons)[2]	6	12	18

[1]Women who are pregnant or breastfeeding, teenagers, and young adults to age 24 need three servings.
[2]Recommendations for total fat and added sugars are suggested upper limits.
Source: USDA, CNPP, 1996.

A careful look at the Food Guide Pyramid recommendations will reveal that it might be difficult to get the amount of unsaturated fat that seems to confer a reduced risk of heart disease. The Pyramid tells us to use fats and oils "sparingly" and does not offer any specific guides to the different kinds of fat. In addition, if the average business person does not choose wisely from the Grain group, they will very likely not reach the desired amount of fiber each day and may over eat carbohydrates and risk getting more than 60% of their total calories from that type of food energy source. These criticisms have been leveled at the USDA in recent years by several leaders in nutritional health. The science behind these criticisms has helped to fuel the renewed interest in the very low carbohydrate diets that have become so popular.

In my opinion, these diets are simply not necessary for eating well and promoting health. They limit our ability to really thrive, which of course includes enjoying all kinds of food. Is that lasagna your mother makes "bad" for you? Is the cake at your daughter's birthday party "unhealthy?" Of course not! Should you never again eat bread? Ridiculous. Diets that say so shift the responsibility of eating well away from the individual and prescribe a dietary pattern that is not realistic, is extremely confining, and for some downright punishing.

Having said that, you need to be cautious about the tendency to oversimplify the Food Guide Pyramid recommendations into "carbs" and "fats." If you do, then you WILL over eat carbohydrates—and these will likely not be the kind of carbohydrates that we know promote health. Considering the specific food group recommendations, we see that, for a diet containing 2200 calories, it is recommended you eat four servings of vegetables and three servings of fruit per day. When was the last time you actually did that for more than two days in a row? If you are like most Americans, you very likely cannot recall. Instead, if your diet is typical, you got your carbohydrates from white bread, white rice, cereals low in fiber, "low fat" foods that contained high fructose corn syrup and trans-fat, and beverages that included 10 to 12 teaspoons of sugar, all the while being very "careful" to avoid the "fat" in foods.

With the values determined through the calculation steps, I recommend a few guides about what and how much to eat.

1) Establishing a goal of 7 to 10 servings (not portions) of fruits and vegetables per day.

That kind of fruit and vegetable intake will look something like this:

1 cup vegetable juice	1 serving
2 cups lettuce in salad	2 servings
1 cup green beans	2 servings
1 banana	1 serving
1 apple	1 serving
1 cup grapes	1 serving

The caloric value of all that food is relatively low: about 400 kcal. If 55% of your 2200 kcal comes from carbohydrates, you have about 800 more kcal that can come from that food energy source. But there are several other important benefits.

First, there are about 14 grams of dietary fiber in this food. Eating whole grain products such as a high fiber cereal and eating two servings of beans will easily get you to the desired amount of daily fiber.

Second, these food choices are rich sources of Vitamin C, Vitamin E, and beta-carotenes, which are vitamins that act as *antioxidants* in the body. Antioxidants are compounds that oppose the inflammatory and tissue damaging effects of the natural products of metabolism. Diets containing foods that are rich in antioxidants have been associated with dramatically lower risk of heart disease. The American Heart Association strongly recommends consuming a balanced diet "with emphasis on antioxidant rich fruits and vegetables and whole grains" and favors this approach over taking pill supplements of these compounds.

Third, fruits and vegetables are the primary natural source of dietary folate, a B vitamin important in formation of red cells and fetal nervous system development. Recommended daily amounts of folic acid, the synthetic form of dietary folate, is 400 mcg per day for healthy adults and 600 mcg per day for pregnant or lactating women. Since 1998, the FDA has ordered that nearly all grain products be fortified with folic acid, so now it is not too difficult to reach the recommended daily amounts.

Finally, eating this amount of fruits and vegetables daily amounts to a lot of eating! Consuming this much food in the form of fruits and vegetables will likely lead to a sense of satiety earlier than consuming simple carbohydrates, possibly because the fiber slows gastric emptying and delays the absorption of sugars and starch found in these foods. This effect can serve to limit total daily caloric consumption.

2) Get enough unsaturated fat.

For a diet of 2400 kcal per day, 25% of total calories coming from unsaturated fat will mean about 65g of unsaturated fat per day. The trick is to get this amount of fat and not exceed your saturated or trans-fat goals. Since most fat containing foods contain a mixture of saturated and unsaturated fat, this will take discrimination.

In an effort to simplify your choices, I encourage you to do the following.

Living Longer Working Stronger

A) Try to get at least three servings of fish per week into your diet.

Fish, especially "fatty" fish like salmon and swordfish, have relatively high amounts of unsaturated fat relative to saturated fat. The unsaturated fats contain omega-3 fatty acids, which may have a role in prevention of coronary heart disease.

B) Use nuts as a snack several times a week.

Nuts are high in monounsaturated fats, and when this kind of fat replaces carbohydrates in the diet, it can raise your HDL and lower your LDL. Nuts also contain fiber and protein, which most carbohydrate snacks are lacking. Nuts are high in calories, about 160-200 kcal per ounce, so it is important to keep track of your portion size. Here are rough estimates of the fat breakdown in a single serving, or ounce of some favorite nuts.

Nuts (1 oz)	Saturated fat (g)	Unsaturated fat (g)	# of nuts in one oz.
Cashews (medium)	2.6	13.2	18
Almonds	1.4	14.6	24
Walnuts	1.0	16.0	14
Mixed nuts	2.5	16.0	18
Macadamia	3.1	21.0	12

Purchase unsalted nuts that are dry-roasted, not oil roasted, which will minimize salt and other oil content. You may have to go to a health food store to get nuts prepared this way.

So a couple of handfuls of nuts a day will give you about 400-500 kcal, about 5g of saturated fat and about 35g of unsaturated fat. Two large epidemiologic studies linked this kind of nut eating with a 30-50% reduction in coronary heart disease incidence and mortality. So exchanging carbohydrate snacks with nut snacks appears to be a healthy choice, as long as you are conscious of the total caloric contribution of this kind of snack to your diet. (Hu FB, Stampfer MJ, et al. Frequent nut consumption and risk of coronary heart disease in women: prospective cohort study. BMJ 1998; 317(14): 1341-1345. and Fraser GE, Sabate J, et al. A possible protective effect of nut consumption on risk of coronary heart disease: the Adventist Health Study. Arch Intern Med. 1992152:1416-1424.)

Increase the use of canola oil and olive oil. These oils—like all oils—are 100% fat, but again the fat mostly comes from unsaturated fats, including monounsaturated and polyunsaturated fats. Use canola oil in place of butter for cooking and baking. Canola oil in particular is a good source of the essential fatty acid alpha-linolenic acid. Many margarines are made from canola oil, but if it is "stick margarine" it has been "partially hydrogenated" and is now high in trans-fat. Choose margarines that are soft and don't have the trans-fat code words on the ingredients. Replace creamy salad dressings with oil-and-vinegar types and add olive oil to pasta and bread instead of butter. A recent study of a cohort of women, those who had a more frequent consumption of oil-and-vinegar salad dressing had a significantly lower risk of fatal coronary heart disease. (Hu FB, Stampfer MJ, Manson JE, et al. Dietary intake of alpha-linolenic acid and risk of ischemic heart disease among women. Am J Clin Nut. 1999; 69:890-897.) Calories are an issue for your total daily needs: Canola and olive oil have roughly 120 kcal per tablespoon.

Using these "replacement strategies" will increase the unsaturated fat in your diet and should decrease the total carbohydrate intake in your diet, changes that have now repeatedly been shown to improve the risk of coronary heart disease, the leading cause of death in our country.

Let's review the strategies I've proposed thus far then see how we might return to the recommendations in the Food Guide Pyramid.

1) Calculate your total daily caloric need.
2) Determine the number of grams of saturated and unsaturated fat that are your daily limits.
3) Aim for 7 to 10 servings of fruits and vegetables per day.
4) Approach your fat targets by eating fish, nuts, and oils in the recommended amounts.

Let's Move on to the Dairy Group.

The Food Guide Pyramid recommends two to three servings daily. The most important argument nutritionally for this recommendation is to achieve dietary goals of calcium intake.

Calcium

Until the age of about 30 years our bones are building density. One measure of bone density is the amount of calcium currently stored in the bones. There are many determinants of bone strength, including genetics and hormone levels, but we know that both physical activity and dietary factors are important. Advanced age puts one at risk for loss of bone density, which can be severe and lead to osteoporosis, a condition characterized by thin bones subject to fracture with even minor trauma. These include spinal fractures, which lead to loss of height, postural disturbance, and other physical limitations, as well as hip fractures, which can be so debilitating and lead to so many other problems that the mortality rate at one year after a hip fracture is as high as 25%. For women there is often a precipitous drop in bone density after menopause, when circulating hormone levels that promote bone density fall. To insure adequate bone density formation and to minimize the potential loss associated with age, adequate intake of calcium and Vitamin D is absolutely necessary. The current recommended adequate daily intake of calcium is 1000mg for adults ages 19 to 50 and 1200mg after age 50.

Most Americans do not get this amount of calcium in their diets. The chief dietary source of calcium is dairy products. There are about 200mg of calcium in one ounce of cheese, 300mg in an 8 oz glass of milk, and about 400mg in one cup of yogurt. Store-bought orange juice is frequently fortified with calcium, as are many grain products, such as breads and cereals. If may be difficult to reach 1000-1200mg daily if you cannot tolerate dairy products. A dietary supplement may be necessary. Nondairy sources of calcium include dark green leafy vegetables, tofu and other soy-bean products, as well as nuts.

Dairy products, of course, contain calories, including carbohydrates (in the form of lactose, a sugar), protein, and fats. Milk and cheese can be relatively high in fat, but today there are readily available low-fat alternatives that maintain the protein or calcium content. Whole milk has about 8 gm of fat per cup, 2% milk has 5, and 1% has 3. Nonfat milk has virtually no fat per cup.

Cheese is a favorite food in the American diet and one of the few kinds of food considered very desirable as a component of all three meals and snacks. An ounce of cheese is the size of about four dice or a slice the size of a computer disc. The Table below provides estimates of the caloric and fat content of various kinds of cheeses.

Cheese (1 oz)	Total Fat (g)	Sat Fat (g)	Kcal
Swiss	8	5	100
Provolone	8	5	100
Cheddar	9	6	110
Mozzarella	6	4	80
Parmesan (3 tbsp, grated)	7	5	75
Part-skim Mozzarella	5	3	65

Eating well should not mean avoiding cheese. Like all foods, the issue is about quantity and frequency, with the knowledge that helps you make deliberate choices. Two slices of provolone on a sandwich is adding about 200 calories and about 10g of saturated fat. In a 2400 kcal diet, that represents about one-half of your target limit of saturated fat for the day. But again, think of those targets as averages over the course of the week and it will add considerably to your ability to make your choices variable.

Red Meat

For many reasons, including availability, price, and possibly health concerns, the average amount of red meat eaten per person in this country is on the decline. (Though our average annual per capita consumption of beef in 1999 was over 65 lbs.) Meat in general is an important source of dietary protein—lean cuts of beef, poultry, and fish all have about the same amount. The chief difference between them nutritionally is in dietary fat. All meat has fat content: Most of it is unsaturated fat, but the amount of saturated fat to total fat can change substantially depending on what kind of meat (beef, chicken, turkey) and where the meat comes from on the animal. In the case of beef, that variation depends on the "cut," and in terms of poultry it depends on whether the meat comes from the breast (white meat) or leg/thigh (dark meat). An additional factor for poultry is the skin, which can substantially change the fat content of a serving of chicken.

The Table below shows the nutritional content of various cuts and preparations of red meat compared to poultry and some fish, for a cooked serving of 3 ounces, which is about the size of a deck of cards. That serving size is in many cases small compared to the usual portion sizes of meat we eat. A "quarter pounder" is 4 ounces, for example. You will notice that for beef, there is substantial variation in the amount of total and saturated fat depending on the "cut" of beef or whether, in the case of ground beef, fat was removed during preparation. In the case of chicken, eating the skin doubles the fat content per serving, as does eating dark meat (from the thigh). Turkey breast is extremely "lean" and has a negligible fat content. *Ground* turkey is typically not very lean, having more calories and fat content than the equivalent amount of a T-bone steak. No type of meat has any carbohydrate or fiber content.

I suggest the following when considering meat in your efforts to eat well. First, it just makes sense to try to eat lean cuts of beef whenever possible and to use lean (90% or 95%) ground beef when preparing meals to minimize total and saturated fat intake. Secondly, cook with, but do not eat the skin of chicken, and realize that eating dark chicken meat is like eating a less than lean cut of beef in terms of fat content. Aim for, when averaged across a week, no more than two servings per day of chicken breast, one serving per day of red meat or dark poultry meat. *Realize that these values are servings of 3 oz, which is less than a quarter pound.*

Following these recommendations will not eliminate meat from your diet. But when combining these recommendation with the recommendation of eating fish at least three times a week, you can see that there will obviously be days when very little meat is eaten and that frequently no red meat will be eaten. Limiting red meat consumption and increasing fish consumption in your diet will make you eat other protein sources, such as nuts (which have the added benefit of being rich in monounsaturated fatty acids) and beans (which have the added benefit of being rich in fiber).

Example: (If our goal for protein in our diets is about 15% of total calories, and our saturated fat goal is no more than 7%, a quick assessment will give us a rough idea of how much meat or chicken you can allow yourself. In a 2400 kcal/day diet, you would not want to exceed 20g of saturated fat per day and your protein goal would be 90g. If you eat a 6 ounce T-bone steak, that's approximately 350 kcal, 6g of saturated fat, and 50g of protein. That's about one-third of your saturated fat allotment and over half of your protein goal.)

Nutrient Comparisons of Meat, Poultry and Seafood

	CALORIES	TOTAL FAT (g)	SATURATED FATTY ACIDS (g)	CHOLESTEROL (mg)	PROTEIN (g)	IRON (mg)	ZINC (mg)
Daily Value*	2000	65	20	300	50	18	15
Lean Cuts of BEEF							
Top Round, broiled	153	4.2	1.4	71	26.9	2.4	4.7
Eye Round, roasted	141	4.2	1.5	59	24.6	1.7	4.0
Mock Tender Steak, broiled	136	4.7	1.6	54	22.0	2.5	6.6
Shoulder Pot Roast (boneless)	147	5.7	1.8	60	22.4	2.6	5.4
Round Tip, roasted	157	5.9	2.0	69	24.4	2.5	6.0
Shoulder Steak (boneless), braised	161	6.0	1.9	80	24.9	3.2	6.7
Top Sirloin, broiled	166	6.1	2.4	76	25.8	2.9	5.5
Bottom Round, roasted	161	6.3	2.1	66	24.5	2.7	3.9
Top Loin, broiled	176	8.0	3.1	65	24.3	2.1	4.4
Tenderloin, broiled	175	8.1	3.0	71	24.0	3.0	4.8
T-Bone Steak, broiled	172	8.2	3.0	48	23.0	3.1	4.3
Tri-Tip, roasted	177	8.2	3.0	70	24.0	3.2	4.2
CHICKEN							
Chicken Breast (with skin), roasted	167	6.6	1.9	71	25.3	0.9	0.9
Chicken Breast (skinless), roasted	140	3.0	0.9	72	26.4	0.9	0.9
Chicken Thigh (with skin), roasted	210	13.2	3.7	79	21.3	1.1	2.0
Chicken Thigh (skinless), roasted	178	9.2	2.6	81	22.0	1.1	2.2
TURKEY							
Turkey Breast (skinless), roasted	115	0.6	0.2	71	25.6	1.3	1.5
Turkey, Whole (with skin), roasted	146	4.9	1.4	89	24.0	1.7	2.5
GROUND MEAT							
Ground Beef, 95% lean/5% fat, pan-broiled	139	5.0	2.2	65	21.9	2.4	5.5
Ground Beef, 90% lean/10% fat, pan-broiled	173	9.1	3.7	70	21.4	2.4	5.4
Ground Beef, 85% lean/15% fat, pan-broiled	197	11.9	4.7	73	20.9	2.3	5.3
Ground Turkey, cooked	200	11.2	2.9	87	23.3	1.6	2.4
SEAFOOD							
Orange Roughy, dry heat	76	0.8	0.0	22	16.0	0.2	0.8
Halibut, dry heat	119	2.5	0.4	35	22.7	0.9	0.5
Tuna, Yellowfin, dry heat	118	1.0	0.3	49	25.5	0.8	0.6

U.S. Department of Agriculture, Agricultural Research Service, 2002. USDA Nutrient Database for Standard Reference, Release 15. Nutrient Data Laboratory homepage **www.nal.usda.gov/fnic/foodcomp**. All beef cuts 1/4" trim, separable lean only, except Tri-Tip, Tenderloin and Tender Steak, 0" trim. All products 3 oz. cooked servings.
*Based on 2000 calorie intake for adults and children 4 or more years of age.

Alcohol

A frequent source of "hidden" calories—calories that many people either don't usually "count" or of which they are not aware, is alcohol. A 12-oz beer is typically about 150 kcal. A "lite" beer is usually about 100 kcal. A glass of wine (5 oz) and 1 ½ oz of liquor is about 90 kcal. These are carbohydrate calories and need to be considered when assessing your total caloric intake.

Several years ago, there was a surge in media coverage regarding wine consumption and reduced risk of heart disease. This attention was the result of epidemiologic studies which concluded that the mortality rate from coronary heart disease in France, where individuals, on average, drink wine more frequently, is about half the rate in the United States despite diets that included roughly the same amount of fat. Further evaluation of this data has led researchers to conclude that the reduction in risk cannot be explained entirely by wine consumption, but there are many studies, (the American Heart Association cites over 60) that suggest a lower risk of mortality from heart disease with consumption of one to two drinks per day of an alcoholic beverage. It appears that no single type of alcoholic beverage—wine, beer, or liquor—confers any greater benefit than the other. Research suggests that the reduced risk of coronary heart disease related to alcohol intake is in part due to its effect on raising HDL (good cholesterol) levels and making blood less likely to clot.

However, the American Heart Association falls short of recommending moderate drinking (one or two drinks per day) to reduce heart disease risk for several reasons. The epidemiologic data that demonstrates a reduced rate of death from heart disease at moderate drinking levels shows an increased mortality rate (from all combined causes) with drinking higher amounts of alcohol. Higher amounts of daily alcohol intake increase the risk of developing hypertension and stroke and may increase breast cancer risk. In addition, prescribing drinking is risky. There are approximately 100,000 deaths annually in this country attributable to alcohol misuse and the lifetime prevalence of alcoholism is about 10%. Usually it is not possible to predict who will become a problem drinker. The American Heart Association recommends that "alcohol use should be an item of discussion between physician and patient." I couldn't agree more.

Weighing the risk and the benefits, I recommend the following. If you do not routinely drink alcohol, there is simply not enough compelling evidence to recommend that you start now in order to improve your health. The other recommendations in this book will provide you with much greater benefit and virtually no risk. If you do regularly drink, limit your intake to one drink a day if you are a woman or over age 65, and two drinks per day if you are a man under 65. That level of alcohol intake is considered moderate and may very well reduce your risk of coronary heart disease. If you routinely drink more than that amount, then you may be at risk for alcohol-related problems.

Losing Weight

This is not a book about weight loss, but if you are overweight and want to lose weight the information provided here can help you. Following the recommendations in this chapter for eating well is absolutely necessary, if for no other reason than they provide a framework for determining how many calories you actually need, depending on your age, sex, and activity level. But no real weight loss will occur over time without applying the steps of critical reflection and physical activity. As we discussed in the beginning of this chapter, eating is behavior, the product of the complex interplay between our thoughts, bodies, and emotions. Like most behavior, it is patterned and usually played out without much conscious thought. Weight loss and weight maintenance requires deliberate, sustained choices, many of which have at first glance little to do with food, but rather are overwhelmingly linked to our emotional lives and the beliefs we have about ourselves and our environment.

An example from my own practice will help. Sarah is a 28-year-old social worker, who has struggled with being overweight since her adolescence. She is bright, well educated, very empathic and insightful into most matters of her life. I have been seeing Sarah for several years now, and we have frequently discussed her weight. I have prescribed a lower calorie diet, better food choices, and exercise. She often leaves our office visits determined to make changes, but when I see her several months later, she has usually gained a few pounds. Sarah is aware that much of her eating is "binge" eating: mid-evening and weekend eating of junk food in large amounts, which she recognizes as a behavioral response to feeling anxious, lonely, or depressed; behavior she finds difficult to control. Over time, we discerned that her mood was more often depressed than not and decided to begin an antidepressant medication. Sarah had a very significant response to the medication, with a mood that was much better, a feeling of being in more control, and the desire to engage in more pleasurable activities. She was also interested in resuming weight loss efforts. I asked her to share with me her self-perceived barriers to losing weight. She began relating things like not knowing enough about food, not having time to exercise, not having enough money to join a gym, etc. But she then interjected another barrier, which she nearly brushed over: "And I don't cook, so that is a real problem," she said, implying that not preparing her own meals forced her to eat fast food and packaged, high-fat, high-caloric foods. She then began listing a few other things. I interrupted her and asked her to stop and consider her statement, "I don't cook."

This was not an excuse. This was a belief—a fixed thought about herself and her abilities. I told her that simply saying "I don't cook" didn't make sense to me. Of course she could cook: She is smart, has a kitchen in her apartment, and has an Italian mother and grandmother who are local and have cooked all their lives. Sarah was taken aback by my directness and my challenge of her belief. She acknowledged all of my points intellectually, but looked at me with a hint of distress. I probed further: "How do you feel when you say 'I don't cook'?" She thought for a moment and said that she felt childlike, somewhat helpless. She said that the thing that comes to mind when she considers the statement is her grandmother telling her that the reason she "doesn't have a man" is because she doesn't cook. That led to more emotions of loneliness.

Here we see the interplay between thought/beliefs and emotions, resulting in behaviors that, for Sarah, include making unhealthy choices about food. The physicality of food, the stimulation of eating, and the sensation of fullness with eating a lot, are the body's participation in the interplay between thought/beliefs and emotions. This is but one example of Sarah's probable multiple layers of patterned behaviors associated with eating and being overweight. Without this kind of critical reflection, which now needs to be, in my opinion, guided and ongoing with psychotherapy, Sarah's prospects for losing weight and maintaining that weight loss are not good.

Many weight-loss programs consider critical reflection to be an important part of weight management. The most common means of initiating this kind of reflection is to keep a food diary. The food diary should have at least four components. First, write down everything you eat, including size and quantity, along with the time of day or night. Second, record what you were doing just before eating, what you were doing when you were eating. Third, record your thoughts that led to your eating, including any thoughts about the foods you chose to eat. And fourth, record your feelings while eating.

Keeping such a log of your thought, emotions, and behavior is not easy and takes time, but if you are overweight or obese, and have not been successful in losing weight and keeping it off, and are frustrated by that experience of repeated failure, then this kind of critical reflection is absolutely necessary. To start, take two week days and one weekend day. You will see patterns emerge in your eating, particularly in your non-meal oriented eating. Those patterns can be changed with guided critical reflection. Recognizing those patterns is the first step to making deliberate, sustained, choices for healthy living.

Prescription for weight loss:

1) Critical reflection: start with food diary, consider psychotherapy
2) Regular physical activity as defined in Chapter Y.
3) Determine goal weight.
   a. Begin by using BMI chart (page 48) to determine weight that is under BMI of 25.
   b. If you are more than 30 lbs overweight, use goal weight as (current weight – current weight x 10%) to start. Losing 10% of your body weight if you are obese has been shown to provide substantial health benefits, including reduction in blood pressure, cholesterol levels, and the chance of developing diabetes.
4) Use goal weight to determine caloric needs based on equations on page 50.
   a. Creating an "energy debt," i.e., taking in fewer calories than you use of 500-1000 kcal per day will result in a weight loss of one to two pounds per week.
   b. This can be achieved by reducing calories taken in and/or by increasing physical activity. "Moderate" activity as defined in Chapter Y, such as 30 minutes of brisk walking, results in a caloric expenditure of about 150 kcal.
5) Apply the recommendations for eating well provided in this book.
6) Other recommendations for weight loss.
   a. Eat three meals a day. Do not skip meals, especially breakfast. Studies show that when people skip meals they overcompensate by eating many more calories than necessary with the next meal.
   b. Add snacks in the afternoon and evening, staying within the caloric goals you have set for yourself.

    c.   Eat slowly: it takes the brain 15-20 minutes to get the "message" that you are full. Eating more slowly will help limit total caloric intake.

    d.   Avoid sugar-containing beverages, such as soda, bottled iced tea, lemonade, and fruit juices. These beverages often contain 200 kcal per bottle and have virtually no other nutritional value. Many people can create a significant calorie debt by simple eliminating these beverages from the diet.

I can confidently predict the success of a prescription very rarely in my medical practice, but if you follow this prescription you *will* lose weight. If you are obese, even a 10% reduction in body weight can result in substantial healthy benefits, including reduction in blood pressure, reduced incidence of diabetes, and improved cholesterol levels. In addition, you will have more energy and very likely more self-esteem.

The Business Lunch (and Dinner)

Many of my business-professional patients relate the difficulty of eating well when frequently faced with meals in restaurants and hotels while attending meetings and traveling. Eating well in this context is difficult, but it too is, of course, simply behavior.

Restaurant food is typically high in salt, saturated fat, and refined carbohydrates. But in my opinion, these are not the real culprits in the diet of the professional whose business obligations puts him or her at the table. Again, the real culprit is the sheer *amount* of food typically eaten in these settings. A restaurant meal that consists of one or two drinks, a few hors d'oeuvres, two or three rolls with butter, a salad with dressing, an entree, and dessert *easily* exceeds the caloric needs of the average business professional in a single meal. If this kind of meal is eaten a few times a week, then weight gain will occur unless a substantial amount of physical activity is added on a regular basis. With this fact in mind, let us consider a few tips for those who frequently find themselves at the table as part of their business lives.

    1)   Plan ahead. Remember to think of your caloric intake across a period of time, rather than getting bogged down in assessing each meal's caloric value. A week is a good interval, because it allows some flexibility to make choices at other times. If a

business dinner is planned, and you know you'll want to partake of the excellent food in a particular establishment, then limit the amount you eat at breakfast and lunch for that particular day, and eat a very light dinner the next.

2) Avoid "automatic eating." On some level, business meals are associated with some level of anxiety, be it from the stress of social interactions or from what is actually at stake from a business perspective at the meeting. In these situations, automatic eating, or eating without thinking (or even enjoying), is very easy to do. Be conscious of the food you decide to eat in these situations, especially the food that comes before the actual dinner. Most people have had the feeling that they are no longer hungry by the time the entree arrives at the table—a sure sign that you are about to overeat!

3) Beware of the bread. Most restaurants serve bread almost as soon as you sit at the table. Waiting to have bread until the entree arrives is a good way to keep the caloric intake down.

4) Avoid "starters." Many hors d'oeuvres offered before the entrée are meals in themselves. Keep this part of the menu out of your routine ordering.

5) "On the side, please." Order salad dressing (preferably vinaigrette instead of creamy) on the side. Typically, restaurants will put nearly three times as much dressing on a salad serving as is necessary.

6) Dessert. Given the extremely high caloric content in most desserts, you may have to simply decline dessert if you must eat out on a regular basis. Again, over the course of a week you will be limiting potentially thousands of calories. If you do get dessert, order a fresh fruit dish or agree to split a dessert with someone else.

These tips can help limit the calories you take in if you eat out on a regular basis.

CHAPTER 9
GIVING YOUR BODY A CHANCE TO REST

At least one-third of adults in this country experience sleep-related symptoms over the course of one year. Most of these symptoms are related to reductions in the quantity and quality of sleep necessary for optimum function, and include, in addition to daytime sleepiness, generalized fatigue, poor concentration, lack of motivation, depressed mood, irritability, reduced productivity on the job, accidents at work, and actual or near miss motor vehicle accidents. Still others may be experiencing the consequences of lack of quality sleep but are unaware of these consequences: They have not developed specific symptoms or may have simply grown accustomed to their state of chronic sleep deprivation.

Lack of adequate quantity and quality of sleep is primarily the result of a few broadly defined categories. The first is lifestyle-related sleep deprivation, wherein businessmen and women are not responding to their cues of needing sleep, are fighting the need to sleep or its consequences, or are sabotaging their sleep with environmental or chemical means. The second category is insomnia, or the inability to sleep at the desired time and for the desired duration. Insomnia is often related to the first category. Lastly are the sleep disorders, which are quite prevalent but under-diagnosed and under-treated. These disorders, which can lead to excessive daytime sleepiness, include sleep-related breathing problems such as obstructive sleep apnea.

As we consider a plan to help us not just survive but also thrive, I would identify lifestyle-related sleep deprivation as perhaps the most important cause of sleep-related symptoms. This kind of sleep disturbance pervades the lifestyle of the peak-performance, highly stressed business professional. Intentional sleep deprivation is an important target for us to take aim at in this book, because it, more definitively than the other causes of sleep-related symptoms, is behavior—behavior about which we can and should make deliberate, sustained choices.

Before we discuss the health risks of too little sleep and the benefits of adequate sleep, we need to learn more about sleep as an important physiologic function.

Though we typically think of sleep as a period of time for our bodies and minds to "shut down," modern science provides evidence that both the body and mind are quite active during sleep. By measuring brain electrical activity and correlating it with other parameters of physiologic function such as heart rate, blood pressure, body temperature, and hormone levels, researchers have mapped out a rather detailed description of what our brains and bodies are up to during sleep.

The sleep-wake cycle refers to alternating periods of being awake and in various stages of sleep. At least two mechanisms play a role in development of the cycle, which includes, at various times during a 24-hour period, a feeling of alertness and sleepiness. The first mechanism is simply the physiologic need for sleep, which results in a drive like hunger, and which is satisfied by a regular period of sleep over a given day. Most adults drift toward a regular balance, or homeostasis, between wake and sleep time over a period of about two days that includes about seven to nine hours per day of sleep. During the course of a 24-hour period, as the person approaches the end of the usual awake period, he or she will automatically get sleepy. The second mechanism is the natural circadian rhythm of bodily functions, in particular the production and release of neurological hormones, which can lead to a sensation of sleepiness or alertness. In general, this mechanism causes an increase in sleepiness twice during a 24-hour period: usually between midnight and 7 a.m. and again between 1p.m. and 4 p.m. The circadian rhythm is influenced by cues, especially external light, and has a 25-hour cycle, which means it needs to be reset daily. For most people most of the time these two mechanisms are in synchrony and lead to our experience of feeling awake or tired. (NHLBI, "Problem Sleepiness in Your Patient", 9/97)

Physiologic changes occur cyclically during sleep and are separated into two different states: rapid eye movement (REM) sleep and non-rapid eye movement (NREM) sleep. Sleep begins with the NREM state, which itself is comprised of successively deeper stages. Stage 1 is light sleep with slow, rolling eye movements and occasionally sudden limb jerks. A person can usually be easily aroused from this stage of sleep, which lasts only a few minutes. You probably have seen someone enter this stage of sleep in a classroom or meeting. The sudden limb jerks can even arouse them back to wakefulness. In Stage 2 sleep, the eye movements become infrequent and muscle tone is usually reduced. Stages 3 and 4 are considered the deeper stages of sleep, and brain electrical activity is manifested by slow waves in contrast to the high frequency waves of wakefulness. It is difficult to arouse someone from these stages of sleep.

Getting through the stages of NREM sleep usually takes one to two hours after sleep onset and then dramatic changes occur: Muscles become paralyzed; heart rate and blood pressure, stable during NREM sleep, are now quite variable, as is the breathing pattern and body temperature. The body has entered REM sleep, named for the bursts of rapid eye movements in this stage of the sleep cycle. The electrical brain activity recorded at this time looks the same as if it were recorded when the person was awake. Not surprisingly, this is the stage where the most vivid dreams usually occur.

After this stage, which can lead to arousal, (if not frank wakefulness), the person repeats the cycle of stages of sleep, though may not proceed through all four NREM stages before returning to REM sleep. During the course of the night, the time it takes to cycle through NREM and REM sleep becomes shorter, and the duration spent in REM sleep in subsequent cycles becomes longer. Typically, the average adult goes through three to five cycles of NREM and REM sleep on any given night and spends 75-80% of sleep time in NREM and 20-25% of sleep time in REM sleep.

Why do we sleep? Science has not provided an absolute answer to that question, other than to study the effects of not sleeping. Given that most physiologic processes (such as blood pressure and heart rate) slow down during NREM sleep and awake-like brain activity occurs during REM sleep, it has been theorized that NREM sleep rests the body and the body's functions, and REM sleep helps the brain or mind to process information. This is a simple, rather mechanistic theory of sleep, but does help to categorize the types of sleep and remind us that both physical rest and "working through" our thoughts and emotions is a necessity.

With aging, several changes occur in the sleep cycle. First, there is a decrease in the total sleep time. Many older adults find themselves awake and well rested at 4 a.m. Second, when asleep, less time is spent in the deeper stages of NREM sleep (stages 3 and 4) and therefore their sleep is lighter, and they can be more easily awakened. Third, there are more frequent awakenings during a given night.

How much sleep do you need? There is no simple answer to this question. On average, when left without alarm clocks, non-sleep-deprived men and women will sleep for about eight to eight and a half hours a night. It is important to note that this is an average value. Sleep requirements are quite variable, especially when age is considered; the vast majority of business people probably need between six and nine hours of sleep a night.

Dr. Kevin Fosnocht

If you reduce the amount of sleep time you need, even by one or two hours over several days, you can accumulate a "sleep debt" and begin to feel its consequences: decreased concentration, irritability, memory lapses, loss of energy, loss of motivation, fluctuating emotions, and decreased coordination. Even a reduction in sleep by one and a half hours of what is needed can result in a reduction of daytime alertness by as much as 32%. One study took healthy young adults and reduced their sleep by 33% of their usual sleep, resulting in about five hours per night for one week. These subjects experienced a decrease in mood, a reduction in psychomotor vigilance, memory impairment, and cognitive and emotional problem solving. (Sleep. 20 (4): 267-70; April 1997) Sleep researchers have demonstrated that many of these consequences can be observed in sleep-deprived individuals *before* they themselves are able to recognize them, and, in some studies, before they consider themselves sleepy.

In a recent study conducted at the University of Pennsylvania, sleep researchers, took healthy, young volunteers and subjected them to a two-week period of four hours nightly sleep. The volunteers took standard psychological and reasoning tests throughout the study period and the results of these tests were compared to results of another group of volunteers who took the test after getting no sleep for more than three nights. Within two weeks the reduced-sleep group had tests results that showed a significant decline in cognitive function, including the ability to multi-task. Their results matched those who had gone three days with no sleep. What's more, the reduced-sleep group reported feeling "only slightly sleepy" even when their performance on the tests was at its worst.

The results of a British study performed in 1999 have special implications for the business executive. The researchers studied healthy subjects following 36 hours with no sleep. The subjects were tested with both standard reasoning tests and a game called Masterplanner, a training tool for managers and MBA students. The main objective of the game is to "promote sales for a hypothetical product and ultimately achieve market dominance and a substantive profit by manipulating various factors." The game encourages innovation for success. After the one night of sleep deprivation, the sleep-deprived subjects did no differently on the standard reasoning tests compared to subjects who got plenty of sleep. But the sleep-deprived group did considerably worse on the Masterplanner game. They responded less appropriately, became increasingly reliant on previously successful decisions (which were no longer appropriate), and failed to produce innovative solutions to an increasingly critical situation." (Harrison and

Horne, Journal of Experimental Psychology: Applied; 2000, Vol. 6, No. 3, 236-249) These results tell us that sleep is important for many aspects of psychological function, especially those which require creativity and innovation.

Other studies have demonstrated that sleep deprivation significantly impairs communication skills. It reduces verbal spontaneity, reduces the ability to "find" words in conversation and debate, and even alters the ability to articulate and enunciate.

What may be even more concerning, given the prevalence of sleep deprivation in our society, especially among professionals, is that sleep deprivation, in addition to having the effects outlined above, also diminishes insight into one's own performance. You may be sleep deprived and not "feel it," and that very sleep deprivation might be impairing your ability to self-assess. This can be hazardous in a position of leadership and in a position requiring definitive decision-making.

Sleep deprivation can have other important health effects. Even a week of partial sleep deprivation (four hours per night), can raise blood sugar and cause an increase in the stress hormones responsible for elevating heart rate and blood pressure. A recent analysis of the data from the Nurse Health Study, which followed thousands of women health professionals aged 45-65 for several years, found that those who slept less than six hours per night on average had a 45% greater risk of developing coronary heart disease than those who got seven or eight hours per night. (Interestingly, women who slept more than nine hours per night also had an increased risk of heart disease.) (Archives of Internal Medicine 163(2):205-9, 1/27/03.) These studies support the idea that sleeping well is linked to healthy living.

Problem sleepiness can become severe: what is called "excessive daytime sleepiness," characterized by the persistent desire to sleep and instances of unintentionally falling asleep at socially inappropriate times (in the middle of a conversation) or dangerous situations (while driving).

Are you sleep deprived? Take a moment and complete this questionnaire, which has been developed to help quantify the level of a person's daytime sleepiness.

THE EPWORTH SLEEPINESS SCALE

How likely are you to doze off or fall asleep in the following situations, in contrast to feeling just tired? This refers to your usual way of life in recent times. Even if you have not done some of these things recently, try to work out how they would have affected you.

Use the following scale to choose the most appropriate number for each situation:

0 = Would *never* doze
1 = *Slight* chance of dozing
2 = *Moderate* chance of dozing
3 = *High* chance of dozing

SITUATION	CHANCE OF DOZING
Sitting and reading	_____
Watching TV	_____
Sitting, inactive in a public place (e.g., a theatre or meeting)	_____
As a passenger in a car for an hour without a break	_____
Lying down to rest in the afternoon when circumstances permit	_____
Sitting and talking to someone	_____
Sitting quietly after lunch without alcohol	_____
In a car, while stopped for a few minutes in traffic	_____
Total Score:	_____

Source: (Johns MW. A new method for measuring daytime sleepiness: The Epworth Sleepiness Scale. Sleep 1991; 14(6):540-5)

If your total score was 1-6, you do not have excessive daytime sleepiness. If your score is 7-8, you might not be getting enough sleep, but you have an average score. If you scored 9 or above, then you very likely do have excessive daytime sleepiness and may have a sleep disorder, which means you should see your doctor and be evaluated.

Sleep disorders are quite common, result in substantial morbidity and mortality, and are under-diagnosed in this country. The major sleep disorders include:

1) Obstructive sleep apnea. This disorder results in the narrowing or collapse of the upper airway during sleep, which causes a temporary cessation of breathing or *apnea*. The apnea causes partial awakenings during sleep time, often not to complete consciousness, but enough to dramatically disturb the sleep cycle. It has been estimated that one in 25 middle-age men and one in 50 middle-age women have obstructive sleep apnea. Symptoms include loud snoring, gasping or choking sounds during sleep, and consequent excessive daytime sleepiness, which over time can cause all the effects of chronic sleep deprivation. One of the most important contributors to the development of obstructive sleep apnea is obesity. A sleep study ordered by your physician can confirm the diagnosis.

2) Restless Legs Syndrome. This disorder causes sensations of irritability, crawling, tingling, or vague discomfort in the legs, which makes the person want to move the legs. The symptoms often occur as one is trying to get to sleep and so interferes with sleep onset.

3) Periodic Limb Movements. Many patients with Restless Legs Syndrome also have Periodic Limb Movements. This disorder is frequently brought to the attention of the person by their bed partners. During sleep, people with this disorder move their arms and legs in repetitive motions, which can cause partial awakening and interfere with the quality of sleep. The disorder occurs more commonly in older individuals and may be present in as many as one-third of people over the age of 60. Diagnosis requires a sleep study.

Depending on the degree of the sleep debt, one night of extended sleep might not be enough to pay back the debt. It may take much longer, even weeks, of adequate sleep to reach a genuine sleep balance.

Dr. Kevin Fosnocht

Problem sleepiness has substantial consequences for our country. Consider a few facts: 80 million Americans report serious, incapacitating sleep problems; approximately 56, 000 police-reported crashes per year result from drivers who were "asleep at the wheel"; and a survey of drivers in New York State found that approximately 25% had fallen asleep at the wheel at some time. The effect that sleep deprivation has on worker productivity and work-related accidents is immeasurably vast.

Not getting enough sleep is unhealthy behavior. Many highly motivated, successful professionals choose not to get the sleep they need. Members of my own profession are especially guilty of this behavior. Most physicians practicing today were trained in settings that asked us to go without sleep for up to 36-40 hours, as frequently as every other night, for months at a time. With this kind of sleep deprivation, we were asked to make complex decisions, communicate effectively with each other and with patients and their families, perform potentially dangerous procedures, and prescribe sometimes toxic medications and other therapies. Needing sleep was considered a sign of being "weak," even unprofessional. Though many institutional changes to provide more sleep are now mandated for physician training programs in this country, these changes still permit physicians in training to be awake and caring for hospitalized patients for up to 30 hours. This is despite the fact that this kind of sleep deprivation—even for one night—can lead to psychomotor performance impairment equivalent to or even greater than the impairment seen in what is currently considered in most states to be alcohol intoxication.

Though we must acknowledge that there truly is a wide variability in sleep requirements, we must each consider our own sleep needs and whether or not they are being met. It can make an important difference between surviving and thriving. Self-imposed partial sleep deprivation is unhealthy behavior, creating a debt that has important physical, mental, and emotional consequences. There is a pattern: behavior expressed by dynamic interaction between our minds, bodies, and emotions, each affecting the other, creating living patterns that usually allow us to survive. There is dramatic interplay between our thoughts about ourselves, our beliefs about what is strong or weak, our emotions, our feelings that we might "waste time" sleeping or anxiety over "missing something" if we get adequate sleep. All this occurs while our bodies are telling us we need rest. Are we thriving? By critically reflecting on these aspects of our selves, we can take steps to change our thoughts, our behaviors, and experience the change in our bodies, with important consequences that can lead to the thriving life.

Insomnia

Insomnia is the most common sleep complaint for which business people, and people in general, seek medical attention. The term refers to the experience of either not enough or poor quality sleep. Usually, people say that they have trouble falling asleep, staying asleep, or both. Sometimes people complain that they wake up too early in the morning with non-refreshing sleep. Often, people experience the consequences of this lack of sleep, which we have described above.

As many as 40% of adults experience some level of insomnia within a given year. For most of these, the problem lasts for a night or two or up to a couple of weeks, then eventually resolves. For others, the problem can be chronic, lasting for at least several nights a week, for a month or more. For those who experience short-term insomnia, the cause is very often some kind of acute emotional or physical distress: concern and worry over a family issue, a major event at work, or a muscular pain or recent injury that makes sleeping difficult. Other causes are more obvious, such as jet lag, a noisy hotel room, or having consumed too much coffee before going to sleep.

For those who have chronic insomnia (poor sleep lasting for a month or more at least three nights a week), the cause may not be very obvious and a medical evaluation is definitely warranted. Many with chronic insomnia have this problem as a manifestation of depression or an anxiety disorder. Others may have a medical disorder, such as asthma, which can get worse at night, or a disorder that worsens with lying down, such as acid reflux, which interrupts sleep repeatedly throughout the night. Many different kinds of medications, both prescribed and over the counter, can cause poor sleep or make falling asleep difficult. Others still will have a primary sleep problem, which careful questioning by their physician will reveal, and appropriate therapy can be prescribed.

For many with chronic insomnia, the issue of sleep itself becomes such a point of concern and anxiety that they cannot relax around bedtime, but rather become focused and obsessive about falling asleep. These obsessive thoughts and anxious feelings need to be dealt with, usually through some form of psychotherapy, to insure successful steps to better sleep.

Though for most people insomnia is transitory and the body eventually adjusts back into a normal sleep pattern, there are several measures you can take to insure the quality and quantity of sleep you need, apart from what we have already discussed, which is to avoid self-imposed partial sleep deprivation. These measures are often referred to as "sleep hygiene" measures, because they are behaviors that promote health—in this case, healthy sleep.

1) Develop a regular sleeping schedule as much as possible, especially waking up at the same time of day. Over time, this sets your internal sleep-wake cycle and can help make the quality of your sleep better.

2) Take steps to keep noise and light at a minimum during sleep time. Though this may go without saying, many people fall asleep to the television or radio or while reading and leave the light on. Though you may be accustomed to these things when falling asleep, if you awake, the visual and audio cues can make falling back asleep more difficult.

3) Avoid extreme temperatures during the sleep period. Circadian changes alter body temperature throughout the course of a 24-hour period, including during the night, especially the early morning hours. Room temperatures that are either too hot or too cold can cause arousals in connection with these natural body temperature changes and interfere with sleep.

4) Avoid alcohol late in the evening. Though a nightcap can sometimes help with sleep onset, it can cause awakenings later in the night, by disrupting the movement through the stages of sleep we discussed earlier.

5) Try not to eat heavy meals close to bedtime (within an hour or two). Heavy meals can interfere with sleep, as your body is working to digest a large amount of food. On the other hand, a very light snack might even help sleep onset.

6) Avoid caffeine four to six hours before bedtime. Caffeine is a stimulant—it can delay sleep onset and disrupt the stages of sleep. I will discuss caffeine in detail later, but for now know that half of any caffeine intake is still in the blood stream four to six hours after you ingest it. Given that it stays in the blood stream for so long, not only does the most recent amount of caffeine ingested effect sleep, but so too does the total daily dose of caffeine.

7) Get regular exercise. (Exercise—again!) Exercise works muscles, relieves tension and stress, and induces hormonal changes that can help sleep onset and the quality of sleep. Because exercise can be activating, it is recommended that vigorous exercise not be done within three to four hours of going to bed, as it might actually interfere with sleep.

8) Use the bed only for sleep (and sex). As we have noted earlier, we are creatures of patterned behavior. On cognitive levels of which we are often not aware, our minds make associations with physical surroundings (our senses) and translate these associations into behavior. Doing work, spending hours watching television, or reading in bed may interfere with the formation of a pattern that includes the bed as a place of sleep (as opposed to leisure). One can train the mind to make this association by practicing the behavior (sleep) in a particular space (the bed).

9) When you are tired go to bed. Again, though this sounds like common sense, too many business professionals who complain of feeling sleepy or fatigued, or who are not satisfied with the quality of their sleep, simply stay up too long. The most common reason for doing so is to watch television. I am not talking about tuning in to a favorite program that interests you and enjoying the show. I am referring to the rather mindless late night channel surfing or watching "anything" until one is actually falling asleep. This behavior does not promote sleeping well. What has happened here, in my opinion, is another example of patterned behavior: watching television (the behavior) is the product of the interaction of the mind (the thought, "I am relaxing" and belief, "television is relaxing") and the body (experiencing the sedentary state and audiovisual stimuli). We get into this patterned behavior often without thinking: it becomes a habit. It is a habit that can seriously decrease the quantity of sleep and very likely interferes with the quality of sleep by providing the brain with thousands of sounds and images at a time when the person should be minimizing stimuli in order to get to sleep.

Source: Sleep Hygiene Measures adapted from "Insomnia: Assessment and Management in Primary Care". National Center on Sleep Disorders Research/National Heart, Lung, and Blood Institute/National Institutes of Health. September 1998

Napping

I am an advocate of napping—even regular napping. Many rely on napping to pay back their sleep debt, which is possible depending on how severe the debt is. If patterned, many can use weekends to take naps and pay on their debt. Sleep researchers have demonstrated that the effects of a night of partial sleep deprivation, including subjective alertness and cognitive performance, can be significantly improved with as little as a 10-15 minute nap in the early-to-mid afternoon (roughly corresponding to the circadian period of sleepiness), with the benefit at least lasting an hour after the nap. Interestingly, a 30-minute nap can make one feel sleepy at first, but within an hour of awakening, equal improvements in cognitive performance are attainable. (Sleep 24(3): 293-300; 5/1/00 and Sleep 23(6):813-19; 9/15/00). Other studies have shown that a nap lasting 20 to 40 minutes in the afternoon can improve mental alertness and efficiency. If one takes into account that subjective alertness and cognitive function are improved with a short nap, then the time taken (15 minutes or so) should not be considered a waste, but rather as an investment in performance. It may be just what is needed before an important meeting.

Caffeine

Caffeine is a drug—a drug many Americans use daily. It is a stimulant, which means it temporarily arouses or speeds up normal physiologic function, such as heart rate and blood pressure. As a stimulant, caffeine wards off sleepiness and it why so many of us use this drug throughout the day.

Only about half of Americans over 10 years of age drink coffee, which is the chief source of caffeine in the American diet, but significant amounts of caffeine are found in other sources, especially tea, soft drinks, and chocolate. You should also know that there are significant amounts of caffeine in some over-the-counter medications—especially certain aspirin containing medications. (Extra-strength Excedrin, for example, contains 65 mg of caffeine, more than what is found in a can of Coke.) The amount of caffeine in these products can be quite variable, but the approximate ranges are as follows:

Coffee (cup/8 oz):   Brewed 60-80 mg
                      Instant 30-120 mg
                      Decaf   2-5 mg

Tea: 30-100 mg
Soft Drink (12 oz):   30-46 mg
Dark Chocolate: 5-30 mg

The typical coffee drinker in this country two to four cups per day. Coffee ingestion has, of course, been affected by the increase in portion sizes, as a "tall" is actually the "small" at many coffee shops.

Caffeine is absorbed into the blood stream and usually reaches peak concentrations about 30 to 60 minutes after ingestion. At least half of a single dose of caffeine (e.g., a cup of coffee) is still present in the blood stream four to six hours later, though it can last even longer if one drinks coffee throughout the day.

Caffeine can raise blood pressure and heart rate, usually only be several points, but this elevation can be more dramatic and consequently more dangerous if you have a heart condition or high blood pressure. For that reason, if you have such a condition, caffeine should be limited or avoided altogether.

We continue to use caffeine as a daily drug because it is effective. Caffeine can increase alertness, especially when one is already feeling tired. Regular doses, such as what one could obtain through normal coffee consumption, has been shown to improve performance and efficiency of simple tasks. Caffeine in the late evening can increase the time it takes to get to sleep, and may disturb sleep, though these effects can vary greatly.

If you are having insomnia or daytime sleepiness, consider the amount of caffeine you are taking in each day, remembering that coffee is not the only common source of dietary caffeine. Begin limiting your total daily consumption by avoiding caffeine after the mid-afternoon.

Jet Lag

Many business professionals have to contend with frequent travel across time zones. Since the sleep-wake cycle is dependent on (1) our physiologic need for sleep and (2) the circadian rhythm of hormone fluctuations that contribute to the sensations of wakefulness and sleepiness, rapid travel from one time zone to another can throw that cycle off and cause jet lag. This term refers to a group of symptoms, primarily inability to sleep at the desired time and sleepiness at inopportune times, and a variety of other symptoms, such as headache, irritability, poor concentration, loss of appetite, and bowel irregularities. These symptoms are related to the disruption of our internal clocks which have been trained to keep a certain "time" via behaviors such as eating and physical activity, and environmental cues, especially light and darkness. What's more, we often travel distances requiring flight for special reasons, such as holidays or important business events when we really need to be awake, alert, and feeling well. We want to enjoy our time off with friends or family and we certainly want to be at peak performance when traveling on business. For most businessmen and women, the greater the distance traveled (the more time zones traversed), the worse the symptoms of jet lag. For these reasons, jet lag can be especially bothersome.

What can you do about it? There are many theories and many recommendations, some better than others in terms of evidence to support their efficacy. Strategies fall into two main categories: resetting the internal clock or simply combating the effects of jet lag. Which strategies to employ depend on how long you plan on being away and how close an important event —such as a business meeting—is to the time you arrive in the new time zone.

It takes three to five days for travelers' internal clocks to be reset without any specific intervention. Ideally you would like to give yourself a few days in a new time zone before an important event. Doing so is rarely possible, particularly on business trips, so other interventions can be used.

With enough preparation time, you can help to reset your clock by gradually altering your meal times and sleep schedule prior to leaving, adjusting the timing of meals and sleep in the direction of the expected meal and sleep times at your destination. Employing this strategy takes at least a few days to be effective, which reduces its practicality.

One of the hormones thought to play an important role in the sleep cycle is *melatonin*. This hormone is secreted by the pineal gland, which is located near the center of the brain. Its peak secretion occurs at about 9 p.m. in most people. Several studies have now found that taking melatonin close to the target bedtime at the destination decreased symptoms of jet lag, especially if one is crossing five or more time zones. Melatonin is available in most drug stores and nutrition stores. The optimal dose for both initiation of sleep and prevention of jet-lag symptoms seems to be 4-5mg. Of note, the 2mg slow-release melatonin was not found to be effective. Realize that this product is not regulated like a drug but is marketed as a dietary supplement or herbal remedy. In addition, it should not be used as a sleep aid at the wrong time of the day: Though it may initiate sleep when taken, it can delay the resetting of your internal clock to local time.

If the travel period will be relatively short, and readjustment of the internal clock is not necessary, then simple measures to combat the effects of jet lag can be employed. These include taking naps and using caffeine. A nap prior to an important event can increase alertness, cognition, performance, and communication. If you do nap for this purpose, be sure to leave at least an hour between awakening and the event, since naps over 30 minutes can lead to some cognitive slowing for about an hour after waking up. Caffeine can improve alertness and performance at several tasks in the short term. Realize that both strategies may interfere with the resetting of the internal clock.

Sleep is the forgotten medicine, especially in our culture. Quality sleep can make the difference between surviving and thriving. Over time, too little or poor quality sleep increases feelings of depression and irritability. Lack of sleep can increase physical symptoms, lead to slower thinking, and difficulty in concentration. Being sleep deprived can impair your ability to self-assess, and therefore make any kind of critical self-reflection more difficult. Take the time to consider the amount and quality of your sleep—then take a nap.

CHAPTER 10
BUILDING AN EMOTIONAL BRIDGE

Thus far, we have considered steps to healthy living that probably make sense to you up front: honest self-reflection on our thoughts and emotions and how they influence our behaviors, getting appropriate amounts of physical exercise, eating well, and getting enough rest. All these steps likely ring true as components of a healthy life. In the following chapter, we will explore another step, which will probably require somewhat of an intellectual—and, I believe, an emotional—leap to link it with health. But as you will see, the evidence is in: This step makes a difference—and may be the most important step to take us from simply surviving to thriving.

You will recall that the root word for health is the same root word from which the words "whole" and "holy" are derived. This etymological fact provides a starting point for us to discuss the next step to healthy living: cultivating positive meaning. What do I *mean* by the word "meaning?" In this context, I use the word to denote an understanding of one's significance and purpose in the world. This understanding should be implicit, informing our choices, reactions and daily lives, yet should be able to be made conscious and expressible, at least in part. And though this understanding should be identifiable, it must be dynamic—it must be ultimately alterable—as all of life is dynamic.

Meaning is at once personal and interpersonal. Though every businessman and woman can be said to have an understanding of themselves in the world, their understanding is always informed and shaped by one's relationship to others, just as our understanding of ourselves shapes our relationships. In addition, meaning is often shaped by our environment, especially life events.

■■■

Why does meaning matter? An abundance of literature in the medical and social sciences suggests that life events, particularly those life events that we might identify as stressful, from daily hassles to the death of a loved one, are interpreted in characteristic ways, which seem to play a role in the effects these events have on our health. In addition, if one already has an illness, the course of this illness is influenced by the way it is interpreted by the individual.

How does all of this work? The details have not all been identified and studied, but current thinking on the topic of how life events affect health include a few key concepts that seem to provide the beginnings of what science hopes will be a complete picture one day. Reviewing these concepts will put "cultivating positive meaning" into a context that makes sense, and is, hopefully, applicable to your daily life. We will begin by examining a concept of which nearly everyone is familiar, both in and out of the workplace: stress.

Stress, a term used quite frequently today, is difficult to define. Stress is an experience. It is a mode of patterned interactions among thoughts, physical sensations, emotions, and behavior—the pattern varying from person to person, though less frequently varied from situation to situation in any single person. The term usually has a negative connotation, particularly when used in ways such as "stressful" or "stressed out," when the implication is that the experience is upsetting or emotionally disturbing. We use the word stress to refer to external events, like workload on the job, financial pressures, an illness, or loss of a loved one. Stress can also refer to internal signals, such as pain or other physical symptoms. We also use the word to talk about the state of being stressed—where a situation is "stressful" or we are "stressed out."

For the sake of clarity, I will use the term stress to refer to the subjective experience of "being stressed," and the term "stressor" to refer to those things, both external and internal, that can lead one to become "stressed."

Stressors, at the most basic level, can be understood to be threats—threats to well-being, threats to security, even threats to life. All living organisms are exposed to stressors—some in the most primitive of ways, such as by weather, lack of food, or being the object of prey. All organisms in turn react to stressors, usually in characteristic ways, and animals respond with rather specific physiologic reactions. The physiology of stress has been studied for decades in both animals and humans, and many of the processes involved in the physiologic reaction have been mapped out.

Nearly everyone—more than once—has been in a "near miss" automobile incident: When you almost got in a crash but at the last second either hit the breaks or swerved clear to avoid a crash. Recall what it felt like when a situation like that occurred: Within seconds the heart rate increases, you can feel your chest pounding, the muscles tense, and somehow you reflexively react—without "thinking" per se. These things occurred because the threat of crashing elicited a fundamental physiologic response seen in all threatened animals. This response has been termed the "fight or flight" response, because it refers to the physiologic changes necessary for an animal to either fight to oppose the threat or to opt for flight to avoid the threat. To do either, the heart must pump faster to get blood to the muscles that are tensed for fighting or fleeing, and the body must be prepared to deal with pain. This is accomplished by the near immediate release of hormones into the blood stream, which have come to be called the "stress hormones." These include epinephrine (or adrenaline) and nonrepinephrine, which raise heart rate and blood pressure; cortisol, which affects the immune system and raises blood sugar levels; and endorphins, which act as endogenous pain killers, and which also affect the immune system. This response is a natural response that is not unhealthy—in fact, it is necessary for survival. This physiologic reaction in more primitive times usually resulted in *actual* physical fight or flight in order to maintain survival.

That is not the case today, of course. Societal and cultural boundaries have been developed to restrain both fighting and fleeing. But the physiologic responses to threats—be they external or internal—persist as the result of our biology. When we refer to ourselves as "stressed," we usually refer to an experience that includes these physiologic responses. Today, these responses are to stressors related to work, family, other relationships, financial pressures, and quite often, medical illness. Though the stressors may have changed from those of our primitive ancestors, the physiologic responses have not.

If these responses occur too frequently or for long durations, they can result in adverse health effects, including high blood pressure, coronary artery disease, strokes, gastrointestinal disturbances, increased risk of infection, chronic muscle pain, headaches, rashes, and depression. It has been estimated that well over half of the visits to primary care physicians are for problems ultimately related to stress.

So what does all of this have to do with cultivating positive meaning? The answer lies in another more subtle but very important part of our response to a stressor. Modern psychology and neuroscience has learned that the physiologic response to a stressor is profoundly affected by how that stressor is *perceived* and how one *copes* with it. In my opinion, both the perception of and the ways in which we cope with stressors are grounded in meaning, as we have defined it.

Events in our lives, from simple hassles to major losses, are first *perceived*. That perception is colored and shaped by a variety of factors, many of which seem to be basic qualities of our personality. Our perceptions typically involve an appraisal of the event as good or bad, or threatening or unthreatening. These appraisals are based on some core assumptions about our lives and our abilities.

What kind of assumptions are we talking about? In a study that has now become quite famous, a group of Illinois Bell executives were evaluated during the very stressful period of the divestiture of AT&T then followed over the next 10 years for a variety of health outcomes. The researchers were able to separate those executives who remained healthy from those who developed illness more frequently by looking at certain personal characteristics, which, when considered together, have come to be known as "hardiness." The healthier group of executives demonstrated this hardiness characteristic, which consists of 1) a commitment to self, work, family, and other values, 2) a sense of control over one's life, and 3) seeing change as a challenge not a threat. Hardiness represents a specific type of positive meaning that seems to confer a benefit to health.

In a more recent study (Manning/Fusilier, Journal of Psychosomatic Research, Vol 47.No. 2, pp. 159-173, 1999), researches examined health care utilization of nearly 200 working adults, who agreed to complete standardized questionnaires to assess the degree to which they manifest the hardiness characteristic. They found that those who demonstrated this kind of perception in their lives had fewer health problems than those who perceived events differently. Other research has shown that hardiness is associated with less mental health problems, higher job satisfaction, less burnout, and fewer physical symptoms, while less hardy business professionals have more fatigue and exhaustion.

It should be noted that most of these studies are performed in such a way that it can be difficult to discern if hardiness *makes* you have fewer health problems or if having fewer health problems contributes to your basic assumptions about life events. Though researchers usually try to take this chicken-or-the-egg question into account via statistical analysis, their results are never foolproof, since they are studying human psychology. There are some studies of hardiness that do not show a significantly better health status in hardy people. Other studies have shown that the most important aspects of the hardiness characteristic in predicting health are the commitment and control components.

But hardiness per se is not the focus of our discussion. The point of this kind of research is that the way we perceive events, especially stressful life events, seems to play a role in the effects these stressful life events have on our health. These perceptions are tied very closely to what we have defined as "meaning," a personal and interpersonal understanding of one's place and purpose in life and in the world. Concepts like hardiness are usually defined as personality traits: basic, almost given, psychological constructs of which those who have them are not necessarily conscious.

But can meaning be learned or acquired. More specifically, for the sake of pursuing health, can positive meaning be learned? In chapter AA, we discussed the work of Martin Seligman, PhD, who is perhaps the world's leading expert on this topic. His research has demonstrated that professionals who exhibit pessimistic interpretations of life events, which Dr. Seligman calls "explanatory style," have more depression and health problems than those with optimistic interpretations of life events. In a recent study, 120 college freshmen who were found to be pessimists on the basis of their explanatory style were randomly assigned to two groups: one got an eight week dose of psychotherapy designed to teach optimism, the other group, or control group did not. The psychotherapy group was found to be in better physical health than those in the control group: fewer self-reported symptoms of physical illness, fewer doctors' visits overall, and fewer illness-related visits to Student Health. They were more likely to visit a doctor for a checkup and had healthier habits of diet and exercise.

This kind of research, which has illuminated how our interpretation of events affects health, underscores the importance of cultivating meaning to live well. The concepts we have discussed thus far suggest that personal commitment to the various aspects of our lives, openness to change, and self-perceived control over events, all in some way mediate health effects. Our ability to cultivate these mediators of positive meaning is dependent on many personal historical factors. But assessing our ability to cultivate positive meaning most definitely requires the first step to healthy living: critical self-reflection.

Coping with stress fundamentally translates to behavior. As we have discussed before, behavior is usually patterned and represents the outward, public expression of the dynamic, reciprocal interaction between the mind, body, and emotions. The thoughts, physical sensations, and emotions stimulated by a stressor, which has been perceived in a certain way, lead to and are themselves affected by, behavior to cope with the stressor. Certain coping behaviors are health promoting, because they appear to reduce the physiologic stress response over time. These behaviors include exercise, pleasurable creative activities, relaxation techniques, and meditation. All require deliberate choices to plan, create time, and do on a regular basis. Many find making such deliberate choices difficult—for unconscious reasons, which is why guided self-reflection can open the door to making them a regular part of one's life.

Other coping behaviors are all too common, and have serious health effects, which we have outlined in previous chapters: substance abuse, regularly overdrinking, overeating, smoking, avoiding sleep, or sleeping too much, excessive television watching or time at the computer. These behaviors, especially if done regularly, are usually means of coping with stressors. They are not positive, as they do not promote health, but do just the opposite. They may help one survive, that is, temporarily cope with life's stressors, but they most certainly sabotage any effort to thrive. These behaviors are patterned, usually unconsciously performed, and it has been my clinical experience that interrupting these patterns requires psychotherapy: critical self-reflection.

In addition to these psychological components of human life, there are at least two other related phenomena which have been well studied in the medical literature and which affect both perception of and coping with life stressors. The first is what many might think of immediately when considering meaning: spirituality.

Before we discuss spirituality and health it will be necessary to define some terms. When we use the term *spirituality*, we often think of religion or religiousness. For the sake of our discussion, I will define spirituality as the attitudes, beliefs, and practices that cultivate meaning, which includes the assertion of a value or reality beyond the individual (the transcendent). This definition is intentionally nonspecific. By *religion*, I refer to the historical system of beliefs and practices of a group. I will use the term *religious involvement* as the participation in the practices of a religion.

In the past two decades, the medical literature examining the link between spirituality, religious involvement, and health has greatly expanded. For some, this topic falls into the category of alternative or complementary medicine. For others, it is considered to be more sociology than medicine: interesting reading, but not directly relevant to the delivery of quality health care. For others still, myself included, it represents modern medicine's acknowledgement that meaning matters to health—and that for many, meaning is derived from spirituality and/or religious involvement.

A 1995 Gallup poll found that 95% of Americans believe in God or a universal spirit. Forty-two percent attend some religious function or service at least weekly, and 60% of Americans feel that religion is "very important" to their lives. Another survey found that over 90% of patients regard their spiritual health and their physical health as equally important. Clearly most people in our country have at least some sense of a reality that is beyond themselves. This reality—which is experienced in a variety of ways that are dependent on history, ethnicity, language and culture—we will refer to as the *transcendent*. It is through the experience of the transcendent, an experience mediated by language, culture, history, and personality factors that many develop a sense of meaning. But what does this have to do with health?

There are now over 1,000 studies in the medical literature that have examined whether spirituality or religious involvement is associated with better physical and mental health outcomes, and most show that mental and physical health are better in those who profess spiritual or religious beliefs or who participate in spiritual or religious practices. Most of these studies have been critiqued because modern statistical methods of taking into account things such as riskier health behaviors were not employed in making the connection between spirituality and health. For example, if we compare the health of 100 church-goers to 100 non-church-goers and find the overall health of the church-going population to be better than those who do not go to church, this fact might be entirely explained by the smoking, drinking, and drug-taking behavior differences in both groups. It would be reasonable to assume, for example, that the church-going group as a whole did less of these behaviors, and therefore had better health as a result. The reasonable conclusion would be that church-going by itself had nothing to do with the better health of that group, but that this group was simply less likely, perhaps because of religious beliefs, to participate in behaviors that are known to impair health.

But it turns out that the explanations are not that simple. Many recent studies using modern epidemiological techniques have carefully taken into account such confounding things such as health habits and have still found that religious involvement is associated with better health outcomes. One of the simplest health outcomes to consider, as we have mentioned before, is mortality or the rate of death in a given time period. One of the simplest markers of religious involvement to measure is religious service attendance. Quality epidemiologic studies have now included tens of thousands of people and have found that those who attend religious services regularly and frequently have a lower mortality rate than those who attend services infrequently.

When we consider specific health conditions, we find the same phenomenon. Most of the studies again use religious service attendance as the primary measure of religious involvement. The majority of these studies show that those who frequently engage in spiritual practices, especially public practices such as attending services have fewer heart attacks, better blood pressure, less depression, less anxiety, and better functioning if disabled.

Before we consider the relevance of these studies to our own discussion—the pursuit of healthy living—a few words of caution are warranted. First, not *all* of the studies that have examined religious involvement and health outcomes show better health in those who are religiously involved. A few have shown no benefit. Second, most of the large, quality studies have focused on simple measures such as church attendance as indicators of spirituality. This kind of measure may say little about spirituality as we have defined that term. Third, these studies are epidemiologic studies that compare large groups of people and see how they differ regarding behavior (church going) and health outcomes (mortality rates or chances of having a heart attack). When these studies conclude that those who go to church more frequently have a lower mortality rate than those who attend services infrequently, that is not the same thing as concluding in a definitive way that church attendance *causes* a lower mortality rate. Though the reader might find this distinction subtle, it is very important. Proving a cause in science is very difficult and the issue of spirituality is too complex for scientific studies to achieve that end.

What can we take from these studies? I take their conclusions to support my contention that *meaning* matters to health. Religious involvement is but one expression—and in the studies we have mentioned, a public expression—of meaning: meaning that is at once personal and interpersonal. How religious meaning is associated with better health outcomes is no doubt very complex. But it is likely that spirituality provides a lens through which stressors are perceived and handled. It may be that religious involvement engenders positive thoughts, leading to optimism, which we have discussed as important in predicting better health. Religious involvement might also engender positive emotions, which we know can decrease circulating stress hormones, such as adrenaline and cortisol, which may also lead to better health.

We have said that meaning is at once personal and interpersonal. The interpersonal nature of religious involvement points to another probable mechanism that can explain the health benefits associated with religious involvement: social support and social integration. *Social support* usually refers to the psychological and physical support that one believes one has from others when coping with the stressors of daily living, including extreme stressors, such as illness or disease. Perceived social support affects how we recognize stressors in our lives. *Social integration* refers to how involved one is with family, a network of friends, and the community. Social integration, which includes sharing of feelings with others, asking for help in dealing with difficulties, enjoying group activities, and giving one's time and talent affects how we cope with stressors. Both social support and social integration have been associated with better health outcomes in a wide variety of populations, especially cardiovascular health outcomes. Low levels of perceived emotional support and a small social network have been found, on average, to be associated with at least a two- to-three-fold increased risk in the development of coronary artery disease over time. In addition, social support appears to be associated with lower blood pressure, lower stress hormone levels, and better immune system function.

The discussion above is not a prescription to "get religion" to improve your health. It is, however, a prescription to self-reflect critically and discern whether or not you have a sense of positive meaning as manifested in your thoughts, beliefs, approach to stressors, emotional life, and behaviors. I am convinced that positive meaning can be cultivated, but cultivation implies commitment, regular tending, and effort. Cultivating positive meaning—just like all of the previous steps—requires deliberate, sustained choices, which are dependent on dynamic critical self-reflection. Cultivating positive meaning is perhaps the most important step to truly thriving—though we have also seen it can help us survive.

CHAPTER 11
GOING TO THE DOCTOR: A CASE FOR PRIMARY CARE

Most business professionals think of going to the doctor when they feel ill. Primary care doctors, though they certainly want patients who feel ill to seek medical attention, are especially interested in seeing patients who do not feel ill but who feel generally healthy. Why? Because, as we have mentioned earlier, most of the morbidity and mortality in this country is preventable, if not by following sound medical advice about behavior, then by routine preventive medical care, which we will discuss in this chapter. I am not going to discuss the issue of particular complaints or symptoms that various patients might have and how a physician deals with them. My focus will be on the preventive care in which a patient and his or her physician should be engaged.

Recommendations regarding preventive health care services are made by various organizations, usually after these organizations have rigorously and critically reviewed the medical literature that has examined the value of these interventions. These organizations base their recommendations on the interpretation of studies that have assessed the value of the interventions and weigh that value against the potential harm the intervention could cause. For example, a mammogram can detect breast cancer lesions very early, prompting surgical removal, radiation, and chemotherapy, the combination of which has a very high cure rate. However, because of the technical limits of mammography as a test, it might also detect an abnormality that gets biopsied but turns out to be non-cancerous or benign. Though this conclusion will come as a relief to the patient, that patient had to experience the anxiety and fear associated with a potential cancer and endure a surgical procedure to determine that there is nothing wrong. In fact, *most* abnormalities found on mammograms that require biopsy are *not* cancer. That amounts to substantial harm, given that most women over the age of 50 get routine mammograms and many end up having an abnormality detected that requires biopsy to exclude breast cancer. Most of the recommendations that I will propose regarding preventive health care are identical to those of the United States Preventive Services Task Force (USPSTF), an independent organization comprised of experts in primary care and preventive medicine, who periodically review the medical literature and rigorously weigh the evidence that supports or does not support certain interventions, based on whether they improve health outcomes (such as disease mortality) and whether the benefits of the interventions outweigh the harms.

Dr. Kevin Fosnocht

How often should I see my doctor if I am feeling generally well?

There are no rigorous studies that provide us with a definitive conclusion regarding how frequently a person who generally feels well should see his or her doctor. The USPSTF recommends a "periodic" assessment with a health care provider, but does not go so far as to recommend an actual frequency, such as yearly or every two years.

Having said that, the frequency with which one should get a checkup or routine physical, can be determined by how often one should get certain screening tests for which there *is* a strong recommendation on frequency, since most of these screening tests require a doctor's order to be obtained. We will discuss these screening tests in further detail. For now, however, my bottom line recommendation for how often adults should get a history and physical, assuming no health problems have been previously identified, is every one to two years. I have purposely given a range of time for this recommendation, since there is no convincing data that suggests any particular interval affects health outcomes. If you are over age 65, however, I strongly recommend a yearly evaluation.

Why every one to two years, even if you feel well? Yes, for several reasons. For one, establishing a relationship with a physician can take time. When I began practicing, one of my first patients, a 40-year-old college professor, said he chose me as his primary care physician because he knew I had just started practicing. I was puzzled by this, and he explained: "I feel well right now. I figure by the time I really need you, I'll really know you." He wanted to establish a relationship with a physician he could trust, so that in the event of illness, that relationship would already exist. He wanted to be able to count on that relationship to weather the storm of illness, should it befall him. (He also said—only half-jokingly considering what little experience I had—that by the time he really needed me I would know what I was doing.) A regular visit with a primary care physician will serve to form a relationship that can prove pivotal once real health concerns emerge.

Apart from the issue of establishing a trusting relationship with a primary care physician, a regular checkup in someone who feels well serves two very important functions. First, the physician can attempt to identify early disease, with which the patient is currently asymptomatic. Second, the physician can perform a risk assessment: a determination of the chances that a person will develop disease over time. No one's risk is static: One's risk of developing a disease changes over time. Not only does it change with age, it changes because one's *risk factors* often change over time. Assessing these risk factors and tracking their change is one of the chief purposes of a checkup. The primary tools of the physician in this context are the *history* and *physical examination.* Let's consider the medical history first.

When a patient has no real complaints upon seeing a physician, it means that the patient a) does in fact have no complaints, 2) is reluctant to tell the physician about certain complaints or concerns, either because the patient is embarrassed by them or does not think they are under the purview of the physician, or 3) they do not consider certain symptoms as abnormal or worrisome enough to bring to the physician's attention. To address these possibilities, the physician will at some point in the encounter ask a series of questions called "the review of systems." (See figure.) The systems refer to the organ systems of the body. Usually the physician will ask direct questions about certain symptoms, ranging from things such as indigestion and constipation to dizziness and headaches. Answers to these questions not only provide clues concerning the presence of early disease, but also get the patient to focus on his or her body; to listen to the signals the body is sending; and, perhaps most importantly, not deny or dismiss these signals when they occur.

We have established in previous chapters that most of the disease burden in this country is attributable to behavior. The medical history taken by a physician asks direct questions about certain behaviors that dramatically affect the risk a person has of developing disease. Most of these important health-related behaviors we have discussed in detail: physical activity, diet, cigarette smoking, alcohol use, other recreational drug use, and sexual practices. Other behavior-related issues we have discussed and which should be part of the medical history include self-perceived stress, work environment, the degree of social connections, and spirituality. Again, not only does this assessment help the physician detect health problems and determine disease risk, but asking patients directly about these behaviors provides an opportunity for basic, critical self-reflection by discussing behavior as an important component of health. Through explicit discussion about behavior, the physician can form a basis from which to offer sound advice about healthy living.

Another very important part of the medical history is establishing a patient's *family history* of disease. Family history is one of the most important contributors to the development of disease: It is an important risk factor for many diseases. The Table X below shows how much a person's risk of disease is increased if there is a family history of that disease compared to someone who does not have a family history of that disease.

Table X

Disease	Increased Risk of Developing Disease
Cardiovascular disease	One 1st-degree relative: 2.0X Two or more 1st-degree relatives: 5.4X
Breast cancer	One 1st-degree relative: 2.1X Three or more 1st-degree relatives: 3.9X
Colorectal cancer	One 1st degree relative: 1.7 X Two 1st-degree relatives: 4.9X
Type II Diabetes	Mother with diabetes: 2.4X Maternal and paternal relatives: 4.0X
Osteoporosis fracture	Mother or Father: 2.0X
Asthma	Mother: 3.0X Mother and Father: 7.0X

Adapted from: Yoon PW, et al." Can family history be used as a tool for public health preventive medicine?", Genetics in Medicine 2002; 4(4):304-310

The family history of disease is dynamic and the physician needs to update continually that part of the patient's history to perform an accurate risk assessment, which is then used to guide decisions about screening, other testing, and even treatments.

After the medical history, the physician usually performs a physical examination. In a healthy adult without specific complaints, the actual value of a complete physical examination is not known. There are parts of the physical examination, however, that should be performed periodically, and these comprise another reason for getting to the doctor on a one- to-two-year basis, even if you feel well. These include:

Height and Weight

This may seem quite obvious, but the importance of tracking height and weight should not be underestimated. You will recall that the best means of estimating total body fat, the primary measure of obesity, is the body mass index, which is determined by height and weight measurements. Given the increasing rates of overweight and obesity in this country, all adults should get these parameters measured and have their BMI determined periodically.

Blood Pressure

High blood pressure, or hypertension, is a leading risk factor for coronary artery disease, stroke, kidney disease, and peripheral vascular disease. It is extremely common—affecting about 43 million Americans—and is more prevalent with increasing age. High blood pressure is a silent disease: It usually does not cause symptoms until it is severely damaging your body, such as the brain or heart. It is estimated that over one-quarter of adults who have hypertension don't even know it. Simply getting your blood pressure checked periodically can identify hypertension. The actual blood pressure value is related by two numbers: the top number, or systolic pressure, which represents the pressure in the blood vessels when the heart has just squeezed out a pulsation of blood; and the bottom number, or diastolic pressure, which represents the pressure in the blood vessel when the heart is relaxing after having squeezed. The values are recorded and reported with the systolic over the diastolic pressures, as in 120/80 (120 over 80). Technically, the diagnosis of hypertension is made when either the systolic pressure is greater than 139 and/or the diastolic blood pressure is greater than 89.

Recent updated guidelines from the National Institutes of Health have reclassified blood pressure values. (See Table below).

BLOOD PRESSURE MEASUREMENTS

Category	Systolic (mm Hg)		Diastolic (mm Hg)
Normal	< 120	And	<80
Pre-hypertension	120-139	Or	80-89
Hypertension	140 or greater	Or	90 or greater

Source: The Seventh Report of the Joint National Committee on Prevention, Detection, Evaluation and Treatment of High Blood Pressure; National Institutes of Health; NIH Publication No. 03-5233; May 2003.

A new category of blood pressure values has been added, called prehypertension. This addition has important public health implications because it includes values of systolic blood pressures in the 120s and diastolic blood pressures in the 80s. These values were previously considered to be "high normal" values. However, analysis of epidemiological data strongly suggest that adults with blood pressure values in the prehypertension range are at *twice* the risk of developing blood pressure as those with lower values. (Vasan RS, Larson MG, Leip EP, et al. Assessment of frequency of progression to hypertension in nonhypertensive participants in the Framingham Heart Study: A cohort study. *Lancet.* 2001;358:1682-6.) In addition, adults over age 40 with a systolic blood pressure of 135 mm Hg have twice the risk of developing cardiovascular disease compared to adults with a systolic blood pressure of 115. Due to this dramatic increase in risk even with small elevations in blood pressure, the National Institutes of Health is recommending lifestyle interventions in all adults who have blood pressures in the prehypertension range. (Lewington S, Clarke R, Qizilbash N, et al. Age-specific relevance of usual blood pressure to vascular mortality: A meta-analysis of data for one million adults in 61 prospective studies. *Lancet.* 2002;360:1903-13.)

The height, weight, and blood pressure are often obtained by a nurse in a physician's office, which is perfectly appropriate. If an abnormal blood pressure is obtained, it should be repeated by the physician.

After these vital signs are obtained, the physician will typically perform a complete physical examination. This may include an examination of the eyes, ears, nose, and mouth; checking the neck for lymph nodes or thyroid gland abnormalities; listening to the lungs and heart; inspecting the skin; feeling the abdomen for enlargement of organs; examining the joints of the body, and checking strength and reflexes. There is little scientific data to support a recommendation that so extensive an examination is necessary on a routine basis in adult patients with no symptoms or physical complaints, which means that either studies showing a health benefit from a complete physical exam have not been done or those that have been done have proven no benefit.

However, there is little if any potential harm in getting a careful complete physical examination by an experienced physician. I say an experienced physician, because the physician must decide, if he or she were to pick up an abnormality, if that abnormality represents something trivial or something worrisome, which would require further evaluation, usually testing—which in itself can cause harm.

Most experienced physicians have stories of patients who have felt well, but who upon careful physical examination have been found to have very concerning physical findings that were the first clues to serious illness. I have detected skin cancer, thyroid cancer, kidney cancer, valvular heart disease, anemia, hernias, and other illnesses in patients who had no complaints, but whose physical examinations were abnormal. Though these instances and anecdotes do not comprise scientific evidence to support a public health recommendation, in my opinion, a complete physical examination, including some of the details I mentioned above, should be performed every one to two years, even in healthy adults who do not have symptoms or complaints.

Getting a regular check up allows for other important exchanges to occur between doctor and patient. The point of this chapter is not to review the scientific literature that provides evidence for or against certain screening tests, but rather to highlight the means by which you and your physician might identify your risk of developing disease, so that this risk can be minimized, and to detect early disease, which is usually more easily and more effectively treated.

Women

Breast Examination

Nearly one-third of all new cancers diagnosed in women are breast cancer, and in 1995, this amounted to about 182,000 new cases. Detecting early stage breast cancer by physical examination and mammography has been shown to reduce the mortality associated with breast cancer. We will discuss mammography further on. During the physical examination of a woman, the physician will perform a clinical breast examination, carefully examining both breasts by systematically palpating the breast tissue to discern if there are any suspicious lumps or masses in the breast. The American Cancer Society and the American College of Obstetricians and Gynecologists recommend that women undergo a clinical breast examination every year, starting at age 40. Many women have this examination done by their gynecologists as part of their gynecologic evaluations (see below). Others will have their primary care physicians perform the exam.

Pelvic examination, Pap smear, and Screening for Chlamydial infection.

The incidence of cervical cancer, a gynecologic cancer that used to be the most common cancer in women, has dropped dramatically in the last 40 years, owing to routine screening of asymptomatic women with the pelvic examination and Pap smear. The pelvic examination involves examining the labia, vagina, cervix, and the ovaries, with their surrounding structures. The Pap smear is a test that involves taking a tissue sample of the cervix, which is then processed and examined to look for cellular changes suggestive of cervical cancer. It also provides an opportunity for the examining physician to determine if there are any signs of vaginal infection or any abnormalities of the uterus or ovaries. The pelvic examination and Pap smear is recommended *annually* for all women who are or have been sexually active or have reached age 18 by the American Cancer Society and the American College of Obstetricians and Gynecologists. Increasing the interval between Pap smears to greater than one year after two or three consecutive normal examinations is recommended by both organizations as well.

The pelvic examination might also include another sampling of the cervical tissue to test for Chlamydia. Chlamydia, a bacteria, is the most common cause of sexually transmitted disease in the United States. It is recommended that all sexually active female adolescents and women at high risk of infection be screened regularly for this bacteria. "Higher risk" includes women who have a history of prior sexually transmitted disease, new or multiple sex partners, under age 25, inconsistent use of barrier contraceptives, and being unmarried. All sexually active women should discuss screening for Chlamydia with their physicians.

Men

Testicular Examination

Testicular cancer is relatively uncommon in the population of men as a whole but is the most common form of cancer in young men between ages 20 and 35. Currently the only way a physician can detect an early testicular cancer is by examination of the testicles, feeling for abnormalities that suggest a lump or mass. The USPSTF says that the evidence is such that they can recommend neither for nor against regular screening exams. In my own practice, I perform a testicular examination on men with their regular physical examination (every one to two years) until age 40.

Digital Rectal Examination

Prostate cancer is the most common cancer in American men after skin cancer. It is the second most common cause of cancer death after lung cancer. Risk of developing prostate cancer increases with age, especially after age 50, and having a 1st-degree family member with prostate cancer. It is also more common in African-American men. The digital rectal examination involves the insertion of the physician's finger into the rectum of the patient so that the physician can feel the prostate gland to assess its size and determine if there are lumps or nodules present. Prostate nodules suggest the presence of prostate cancer, and feeling such nodules usually means the physician will advise going on to prostate biopsy. Most prostate cancers, however, cannot be felt, either because of their location on the prostate or their size, which means a normal prostate exam does not rule out prostate cancer. The American Urological Association (AUA) says that the digital rectal examination (along with the PSA blood test, which we will discuss below) should be offered to all men age 50 or older, if they have a life expectancy of 10 years or more. By saying "offered," the AUA acknowledges that there is not overwhelming scientific data to support screening all men with no symptoms, especially if the life expectancy is relatively short, in which case, even if the patient does have prostate cancer, he will likely not die from the disease, since it is usually a slow growing tumor. Using the term "offered" also underscores the importance of the physician and the patient discussing the benefits and risks of certain exams. I offer Caucasian men over 50 and African-American men over 40 prostate cancer screening.

Laboratory and Other Tests

After the physical examination, the checkup usually includes the recommendation of other tests. These tests, like the history and physical examination, are designed to 1) detect early disease, and 2) determine if you are at risk for disease, so that the risk can be lowered, if possible. They include:

All Adults

Blood Tests. Cholesterol.

High blood cholesterol is not a disease in and of itself. Rather, high cholesterol is an important contributor to the development of disease, in particular, cardiovascular disease, the leading cause of death in this country. As such, abnormal cholesterol level is a major risk factor for cardiovascular disease. It is also a risk factor that can be modified (unlike age), meaning lowering blood cholesterol can reduce the risk of developing cardiovascular disease, hence the importance of getting it measured. The National Cholesterol Education Program of the National Heart, Lung, and Blood Institute recommends a fasting lipid profile once every five years for adults over age 20. That profile should include a measurement of:

> The total cholesterol
> High-density lipoprotein (HDL) or "good" cholesterol
> Low-density lipoprotein (LDL) or "bad" cholesterol
> Triglycerides.

Glucose

The incidence of diabetes is on the rise in this country and is currently present in an estimated 16 million people, nearly one-third of whom do not know they have the disease. The risk of having diabetes increases with age (especially over 45 years), being overweight, being sedentary, having a family history of diabetes (adult-onset), or a personal history of gestational diabetes. In addition, African-Americans, Hispanic-Americans and Asian-Americans are at a higher risk of developing diabetes than Caucasian-Americans. The American Diabetes Association, therefore, recommends screening for diabetes with a fasting blood glucose ("blood sugar") in all adults after the age of 45 at least every three years. They recommend that physicians should consider obtaining the test at an earlier age or more frequently if the risk factors we mentioned, in particular being overweight or obese, are present. Since even a minimally elevated fasting blood glucose (110 to 125), which would not qualify for overt diabetes, could contribute to an increased risk of cardiovascular disease, obtaining a fasting blood glucose also serves to determine that risk.

Given the prevalence of being sedentary, overweight, and having high blood pressure, and cholesterol, and since cardiovascular disease is the leading cause of death in this country, I order a blood glucose at regular intervals in most of my primary care patients.

Age $\geq$45 years

Overweight (BMI $\geq$25 kg/m^{2*})

Family history of diabetes (i.e., parents or siblings with diabetes)

Habitual physical inactivity

Race/ethnicity (e.g., African-Americans, Hispanic-Americans, Native Americans, Asian-Americans, and Pacific Islanders)

Previously identified IFG or IGT

History of GDM or delivery of a baby weighing >9 lbs

Hypertension ($\geq$140/90 mmHg in adults)

HDL cholesterol $\leq$35 mg/dl (0.90 mmol/l) and/or a triglyceride level $\geq$250 mg/dl (2.82 mmol/l)

Polycystic ovary syndrome

History of vascular disease

Source: Diabetes Care 26:S21-S24, 2003
© 2003 by the American Diabetes Association, Inc.

PSA (prostate specific antigen)

This blood test detects a chemical that is made by the prostate gland. It can be elevated in several conditions, including prostate infections, prostate enlargement (BPH, or benign prostatic hyperplasia), and prostate cancer, which is why the blood test is considered as a screening test for this cancer. Along with the digital rectal examination, it is recommended that this blood test be offered to men over the age of 50 on an annual basis for those men who are considered to have a life expectancy of greater than 10 years. It should be offered at an earlier age to a man with risk factors (such as race or family history of the disease). Again, by saying "offered," it is recommended that the physician and patient discuss the value of the test and what the patient's wishes are regarding how to proceed with a positive, or elevated, blood test.

There are hundreds of other laboratory tests that your physician could order which can detect abnormalities in one or more organs. Most of these are ordered in response to a concern over a finding from the medical history or physical examination. For example, in an older woman with fatigue and a family history of thyroid disease, a thyroid blood test would be indicated. In a patient with pain in the upper, right quadrant of the abdomen, a liver function blood test would make sense. If a patient bruised easily or has very frequent nose bleeds, a blood count and blood clotting tests would be ordered. But for the healthy adult with no symptoms, an unconcerning medical history, and a normal physical examination, there is little value to any other blood tests other than those we just mentioned. There are, however, several other kinds of tests that should be considered.

ECG (Electrocardiogram)

The ECG is a test done in the physician's office which takes a 10-second picture of the electrical activity of the heart. It can detect abnormal heart rhythm (if the abnormal rhythm is occurring at the time of the test) and provide clues as to whether or not someone has had a heart attack in the past, or whether or not the heart is enlarged. In a patient with no concerning findings on medical history or physical examination, and who has no complaints relating to the heart, the ECG will provide little in the way of detecting silent illness. However, the American Heart Association and American College of Cardiology recommend obtaining an ECG in adults over 40 years of age to establish a baseline picture of the heart, so that, if the patient does develop cardiovascular symptoms in the future, an ECG at that time can be compared to the baseline study, to see if a significant change is present that might indicate that the symptoms are indeed being caused by an abnormality of the heart.

Other Tests:

All Adults

Colorectal Cancer Screening

Colorectal cancer is the second most common form of cancer in the United States. Risk factors for colorectal cancer include a family history of colon cancer or colon polyps (in a 1st-degree relative), diets high in fat or low in fiber, or a personal history of endometrial, ovarian, or breast cancer. The highest risk of getting colorectal cancer comes from those with a family history of colon polyps syndromes (e.g., hereditary polyposis), which are relatively uncommon, or those with a personal history of ulcerative colitis, an inflammatory disease of the colon. There is now good evidence that screening for colorectal cancer reduces the mortality from colon cancer. Screening in this case serves two functions. First, it allows for precancerous growths, called polyps, to be identified then removed, before one even gets colon cancer. Second, it can identify early colorectal cancers, which are much easier and more successfully treated. The USPSTF strongly recommends that clinicians screen men and women 50 years of age or older.

There are currently four accepted methods of colon cancer screening. The simplest is called *fecal occult blood testing* (FOBT). This test checks the patient's stool (fecal matter) for the presence of microscopic, or "occult," amounts of blood. The test is done by taking a stool sample at three different times, putting it on a special sample card given to you by your health care provider, and having them use a chemical reaction to detect blood. If the test is positive, it would prompt a more invasive means of looking for colon polyps or colon cancer. Which leads us to the other methods of screening.

A *sigmoidoscopy* involves having a flexible scope passed into the rectum and advanced through the latter one-third of the colon, which includes a part of the colon called the sigmoid colon, hence the name of the test. The physician can visualize this area of the colon and identify polyps or cancers. Some physicians are able to take biopsies through the scope, to sample tissue which can then be prepared and studied microscopically to determine if the type of growth is worrisome for cancer. If one or more polyps are found, the patient must proceed to yet another test, a colonoscopy, to insure that there are no other polyps in the rest of the colon.

A colonoscopy also involves a flexible scope, but this time it is much longer, so that the entire colon can be visualized. This scope is large enough to allow not only for biopsies, but in some cases actual removal of a polyp, which is then examined microscopically for evidence of cancer. A colonoscopy requires sedation with intravenous medicines prior to being performed. Since a colonoscopy, visualizes the entire colon, and the patient is sedated, which means the procedure can take longer without discomfort to the patient, this study can provide a better look inside the colon, allowing for the frequency of screening with this method to be less.

An alternative to colonoscopy is the *double contrast barium enema*. The double contrast is made up of air, which distends the colon, and liquid barium, which can be picked up by x-ray. Radiologists then interpret the x-ray pictures, looking for evidence of abnormal growths in the colon. If these are identified, a colonoscopy would be indicated.

You may be considering the tests above and realize that if the FOBT, the sigmoidoscopy, or the barium enema show evidence of polyps, then a colonoscopy would be necessary for further diagnosis, and possibly treatment (removal of the polyp). Why not just do a colonoscopy? That is an excellent question, and many experts are now recommending just that.

For those 50 years of age and over, the American Cancer Society recommends FOBT annually along with sigmoidoscopy every five years or a colonoscopy every 10 years; a barium enema every five to 10 years could substituted for colonoscopy. Currently Medicare will cover annual FOBT and/or sigmoidoscopy every four years. It will also cover a colonoscopy every 10 years.

Mammogram for Women

We discussed breast cancer earlier. Yearly mammography is recommended by the American Cancer Society and the American College of Obstetricians and Gynecologists. The USPSTF recommends that women get mammograms every one to two years. There has been some controversy regarding when average risk women should start getting mammograms and for how long they should continue. The USPSTF and the American Cancer Society recommend beginning annual screening at age 40. Screening should continue until at least age 69 and continue after that age if they do not have illnesses that will significantly limit their life expectancy. All women should discuss breast cancer screening with their physicians.

Bone-density Testing

Osteoporosis is a bone disease characterized by loss of bone density. The chief medical concern regarding osteoporosis is that the low bone mass can lead to an increased risk of bone fracture, especially of the hip and spinal column. All adults begin to lose some bone density around the age of 30. In women, the rate of loss of bone density can be dramatic after menopause, due to the effects of the loss of estrogen. It has been estimated that about 1.3 million osteoporosis-related fractures occur each year in the United States. Risk factors for osteoporosis, in addition to age and female sex, include Caucasian race, low body weight, family history, and cigarette smoking. Because of the high number of fractures associated with osteoporosis, and because there are treatments which have been shown to reduce the rate of loss of bone density, the USPSTF recommends that women age 65 and older be screened routinely for osteoporosis. Screening should begin at age 60 if they are at increased risk for osteoporotic fracture.

The most widely available means of screening for osteoporosis is the DEXA (dual energy x-ray absorptiometry) scan, which measures bone density in the lower spine and hip and compares the measured density to the bone density of an average young woman. A scale is used to score the patient's bone density and determine if the bone density is low.

Though the DEXA scan is a useful screening test, and there are treatment options for osteoporosis that may reduce the risk of spine and hip fracture, it should be emphasized that preventive measures to reduce fracture risk are important. These include adequate dietary calcium and vitamin D intake, weight-bearing exercise, and, of course, for so many other reasons as well, not smoking.

Immunizations

Immunizations are another important part of preventive medicine. In the 21st century, we take for granted the public health effects of immunization, which have so changed the landscape of disease and illness in this country. Most readers will have undergone childhood immunizations or have otherwise become immune to certain illnesses by actually contracting the disease (such as chicken-pox). But there are a few immunizations that all adults should get periodically.

Influenza Vaccine

Influenza infection, or the flu, is a virus infection that causes severe fatigue, fever, cough and congestion that typically last for several days. A yearly influenza vaccine is recommended for all adults over age 50. It is also recommended for adults of any age who have chronic lung or heart conditions. There are several other groups for whom the vaccine is strongly recommended (see insert). Though a minority of people who receive the vaccine may feel one or two days of achiness or mild fatigue, the flu vaccine *cannot*, contrary to popular belief, *cause* the flu. The influenza vaccine, or flu shot, is developed on a yearly basis to match as closely as possible the potential strains of the virus that might cause infection in any particular year. Flu season is usually October through March, so September or October are good months to get a flu shot.

Pneumococcal Vaccine

The most common cause of bacterial pneumonia is an organism called *Streptococcus pneumoniae*. A vaccine against this organism is recommended if you are over age 65. If you have a chronic medical condition such as diabetes or kidney disease, you should receive this vaccination no matter what your age. Though it is not clear to what extent the vaccine prevents getting infected with Strep pneumonia, it does seem to reduce the chances that the bacteria get into the blood stream and reduces mortality from the infection. A one-time revaccination may be beneficial five to 10 years after the first vaccination.

Tetanus Shot

Tetanus is caused by a toxin produced by a bacterium called *Clostridium tetani*, and its most common presentation is total body muscle spasm and rigidity. The condition can be fatal. Primarily as the result of immunization programs, tetanus is now a very uncommon disease in the United States. Most people in this country have undergone the primary immunization series in childhood, but for adults, a booster shot is recommended every 10 years. The vaccine is produced as a combination vaccine, with a vaccine against diphtheria, now another rare infection.

Hepatitis B

There are several different kinds of viruses that can cause hepatitis, or inflammation of the liver. Hepatitis B is a virus transmitted from person to person via contact with bodily fluids. Infection with hepatitis B can over years result in liver failure or cirrhosis and increases the risk of developing liver cancer. In this country, hepatitis is transmitted primarily through sexual contact and sharing of needles used for injecting drugs. Hepatitis B vaccination is being administered routinely to young adults. For adults over 30, indications to receive the vaccination include the following: 1) persons with more than one sex partner in the previous six months, 2) persons with a recently acquired sexually transmitted disease, 3) men who have sex with men, and 4) health-care workers and public-safety workers who have exposure to blood in the workplace. I offer hepatitis B vaccination to any sexually active adult who is not in a committed, monogamous relationship.

Special Immunizations

For business executives who travel abroad, special immunizations may be recommended. Many academic medical centers have "Travel Medicine" clinics which offer information, counseling, and administration of recommended vaccines. Most of these clinics follow the recommendations for travelers published by the Centers for Disease Control and Prevention. These recommendations are regularly updated and can be found at the following website: **www.cdc.gov/travel**.

Executive Health Programs

Many corporations contract with large, usually academic, medical centers, and offer an executive health program. Such programs typically offer comprehensive interval health assessments for executives, outside of, or in addition to, the company's regular health insurance plan. The health assessments usually include:

- a complete history and physical examination
- age and sex appropriate screening tests
- a formalized, detailed report, made available to the executive's primary care provider, including:
  - test results and their interpretations
  - a formalized risk assessment for the major diseases
  - recommendations for further testing or interventions

You may recognize that these health assessments include nearly every item mentioned above in our discussion on seeing a primary care physician. So how are these assessments different than getting good preventive care from your primary care physician? The short answer is that, taken as a whole, an executive health assessment should *not* be different from that provided by a good primary care physician. But many of these programs offer additional evaluations that can be very valuable and are, as we have mentioned in previous chapters, important in a comprehensive health assessment. These include a detailed nutritional assessment, a careful sleep history, a stress assessment, and appropriate counseling for behavioral change to promote health. Few standard insurance plans routinely offer such expert assessments, so one could take advantage of an executive health program to undergo such an evaluation.

It should be mentioned, however, that many executive health programs offer other services, usually in the form of testing that involves technology, for which there is little compelling evidence to perform routinely in asymptomatic adults. For example, many executive health plans will offer mechanized testing of hearing, even in asymptomatic patients. The U.S. Preventive Services Task Force says that "there is insufficient evidence to recommend for or against routinely screening asymptomatic working-age adults for hearing impairment." It goes on to cite the low prevalence of hearing impairment, the high cost of the testing, and the likelihood that if one has a hearing problem he or she will bring it to a physician's attention if it is of concern. Other examples include the routine ordering of screening chest x-ray, pulmonary function studies, and more advanced (and costly) tests such as total-body CT scanning. These tests have little value in refining health risk or identifying early disease unless indicated by the history or physical examination of the patient. Yet they are often included in the standard package offered to corporations that contract for these programs at considerable cost.

Having said that, these executive health programs offer other advantages. The first is convenience. Most plans include the entire basic evaluation on a single day. Here is a sample schedule for a one-day executive health assessment:

7:15 a.m.	Arrival/welcome to the Executive Health Program by Program concierge
7:30 to 10 a.m.	Comprehensive Health Assessment, including complete history and physical examination by Program physician, electrocardiogram, exercise tolerance test, chest x-ray and lab tests
10 to 10:15 a.m.	Continental Breakfast
10:30 to 11:30 a.m.	Stress Management Assessment
11:30 a.m. to noon	Exercise Assessment
noon to 2 p.m.	Personal time/lunch
2 to 2:30 p.m.	Nutrition Assessment
2:30 to 3:30 p.m.	Exit Consultation, including review of test results from that morning
3:30 to 3:45 p.m.	Program Evaluation
4 p.m.	Departure

Such a comprehensive health assessment would usually require multiple office visits to several different locations, possibly over a few months time. Clearly the convenience of a single day assessment is a real advantage for a busy professional.

The second advantage is more time with health professionals than is typically possible in an average medical practice. This includes time not only with the physician, who will be highly motivated to discuss health issues with you, but also time with a nutritionist and often a psychologist and physical therapist. One's questions and concerns can be answered in a timely fashion.

Thirdly, these programs usually produce a document that clearly outlines the results of the assessment. Such a product serves as a record of one's status by which changes can be measured. In addition, this document can be shared with the executive's primary care physician to help guide ongoing care that he or she provides.

Many academic medical centers, i.e., those associated with a major university, offer executive health programs. These can be accessed via the medical center's website. Here are a few examples:

Duke University
http://www.dukeexechealth.org/(utpwvwadm2gljc452yrgkhel)/EHP/Programs/formen.aspx

University of Chicago
http://www.uchospitals.edu/executivehealth/

Johns Hopkins
http://www.jhintl.net/English/Patients/patientsHealth.asp

University of Iowa
http://www.uihealthcare.com/depts/uiexecutivehealth/

UCLA
http://www.healthcare.ucla.edu/executive_health/index.asp

University of Florida
http://www.exechealth.ufl.edu/packages.shtml

Harvard University
http://www.brighamandwomens.org/patient/ehp.asp

Best Selling Books

Visit your local bookseller today or visit www.Aspatore.com
for retail locations carrying Aspatore books.

Reference

Business Travel Bible – Must Have Phone Numbers, Business Resources & Maps
The Golf Course Locator for Business Professionals – Golf Courses Closest to
Largest Companies, Law Firms, Cities & Airports
Executive Adventures: 50+ Adrenaline Filled Out of the Office Escapes
Business Grammar, Style & Usage – Rules for Articulate and Polished Business
Writing and Speaking
ExecRecs – Executive Recommendations For The Best Business Products
The C-Level Test – Business IQ & Personality Test for Professionals
The Business Translator-Business Words, Phrases & Customs in Over 65
Languages

Management

Corporate Ethics – The Business Code of Conduct for Ethical Employees
The Governance Game – Restoring Boardroom Excellence & Credibility in
America
Inside the Minds: Leading CEOs – CEOs Reveal the Secrets to Leadership &
Profiting in Any Economy
Inside the Minds: The Entrepreneurial Problem Solver – Entrepreneurial
Strategies for Identifying Opportunities in the Marketplace
Inside the Minds: Leading Consultants – Industry Leaders Share Their
Knowledge on the Art of Consulting
Inside the Minds: Leading Women – What It Takes to Succeed & Have It All in
the 21st Century
Being There Without Going There: Managing Teams Across Time Zones,
Locations and Corporate Boundaries

Technology

Inside the Minds: Leading CTOs – The Secrets to the Art, Science & Future of
Technology
Software Product Management – Managing Software Development from Idea to
Development to Marketing to Sales
Inside the Minds: The Telecommunications Industry – Leading CEOs Share
Their Knowledge on The Future of the Telecommunications Industry
Web 2.0 AC (After Crash) – The Resurgence of the Internet and Technology
Economy
Inside the Minds: The Semiconductor Industry – Leading CEOs Share Their
Knowledge on the Future of Semiconductors

**To Order or For Customized Suggestions From an Aspatore Business Editor,
Please Call 1-8_66_-Aspatore (277-2867) Or
Visit** www.Aspatore.com

Venture Capital/Entrepreneurial

Term Sheets & Valuations – A Detailed Look at the Intricacies of Term Sheets & Valuations

Deal Terms – The Finer Points of Deal Structures, Valuations, Term Sheets, Stock Options and Getting Deals Done

Inside the Minds: Leading Deal Makers – Leveraging Your Position and the Art of Deal Making

Hunting Venture Capital – Understanding the VC Process and Capturing an Investment

Inside the Minds: Entrepreneurial Momentum – Gaining Traction for Businesses of All Sizes to Take the Step to the Next Level

Legal

Inside the Minds: Privacy Matters – Leading Privacy Visionaries Share Their Knowledge on How Privacy on the Internet Will Affect Everyone

Inside the Minds: Leading Lawyers – Leading Managing Partners Reveal the Secrets to Professional and Personal Success as a Lawyer

Inside the Minds: The Innovative Lawyer – Leading Lawyers Share Their Knowledge on Using Innovation to Gain an Edge

Inside the Minds: Leading Labor Lawyers – Labor Chairs Reveal the Secrets to the Art & Science of Labor Law

Financial

Inside the Minds: Leading Accountants – The Golden Rules of Accounting & the Future of the Accounting Industry and Profession

Inside the Minds: Leading Investment Bankers – Leading I-Bankers Reveal the Secrets to the Art & Science of Investment Banking

Inside the Minds: The Financial Services Industry – The Future of the Financial Services Industry & Professions

Building a $1,000,000 Nest Egg – 10 Strategies to Gaining Wealth at Any Age

Inside the Minds: The Return of Bullish Investing

Inside the Minds: The Invincibility Shield for Investors

Marketing/Advertising/PR

Inside the Minds: Leading Marketers–Leading Chief Marketing Officers Reveal the Secrets to Building a Billion Dollar Brand

Inside the Minds: Leading Advertisers – Advertising CEOs Reveal the Tricks of the Advertising Profession

Inside the Minds: The Art of PR – Leading PR CEOs Reveal the Secrets to the Public Relations Profession

Inside the Minds: PR Visionaries – PR CEOS Reveal the Golden Rules